FORGET THIS
Chronic Pain
NONSENSE

A pain tracking journal

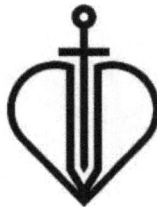

WELLNESS WARRIOR PRESS

Copyright © 2020 by Wellness Warrior Press

ISBN: 978-1-7775422-1-4

This journal belongs to…

_____

DOCTOR / SPECIALIST INFORMATION

Name	Address	Contact

DAILY MEDICATION / SUPPLEMENTS

Medication / Supplement	Dosage

Summary

For each journal entry, return to this summary page and
rate your overall pain / discomfort level
(1 being no pain and 10 being unbearable)

Entry #	Rating	Entry #	Rating
1		31	
2		32	
3		33	
4		34	
5		35	
6		36	
7		37	
8		38	
9		39	
10		40	
11		41	
12		42	
13		43	
14		44	
15		45	
16		46	
17		47	
18		48	
19		49	
20		50	
21		51	
22		52	
23		53	
24		54	
25		55	
26		56	
27		57	
28		58	
29		59	
30		60	

Date: _____

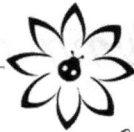

How are you feeling today?

Like death	Terrible	Not good	Meh	Good	Great!	Amazing!

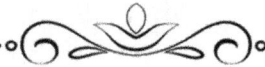

RATE YOUR PAIN LEVEL

(1) (2) (3) (4) (5) (6) (7) (8) (9) (10)

Describe your pain / symptoms   Where do you feel it?

	am	pm
	☐	☐
	☐	☐
	☐	☐
	☐	☐
	☐	☐
	☐	☐
	☐	☐
	☐	☐

Front   *Back*

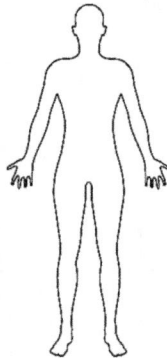

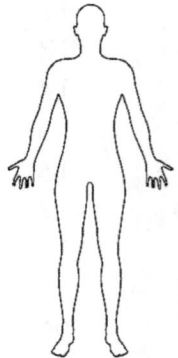

What about your...?   Feeling sick?

Mood	(1)(2)(3)(4)(5)(6)(7)(8)(9)(10)	☐ Nope!
Energy levels	(1)(2)(3)(4)(5)(6)(7)(8)(9)(10)	☐ Yes...
Mental clarity	(1)(2)(3)(4)(5)(6)(7)(8)(9)(10)	

☐ Nausea   ☐ Diarrhea   ☐ Vomiting   ☐ Sore throat

☐ Congestion   ☐ Coughing   ☐ Chills   ☐ Fever

Other symptoms: _____

LET'S EXPLORE SOME MORE

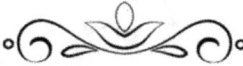

Hours of Sleep ① ② ③ ④ ⑤ ⑥ ⑦ ⑧ ⑨ ⑩ ⊕

Sleep Quality ① ② ③ ④ ⑤ ⑥ ⑦ ⑧ ⑨ ⑩

WEATHER

☐ Hot ☐ Mild ☐ Cold BM Pressure: _____

☐ Dry ☐ Humid ☐ Wet Allergen Levels: _____

STRESS LEVELS

| None | Low | Medium | High | Max | @$#%! |

FOOD / MEDICATIONS

FOOD / DRINKS	MEDS / SUPPLEMENTS	TIME	DOSE

☐ usual daily medication

EXERCISE / DAILY ACTIVITY

☐ Heck yes, I worked out.

☐ I managed to exercise a bit.

☐ No, I haven't exercised at all.

☐ I did some stuff, and that counts.

DETAILS

NOTES / TRIGGERS / IMPROVEMENTS

WRITE ONE THING YOU'RE GRATEFUL FOR

Date:_____

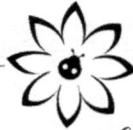

How are you feeling today?

| Like death | Terrible | Not good | Meh | Good | Great! | Amazing! |

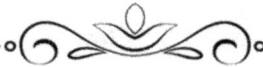

RATE YOUR PAIN LEVEL

(1) (2) (3) (4) (5) (6) (7) (8) (9) (10)

Describe your pain / symptoms

Where do you feel it?

	am	pm
	☐	☐
	☐	☐
	☐	☐
	☐	☐
	☐	☐
	☐	☐
	☐	☐
	☐	☐

Front *Back*

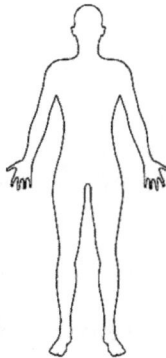

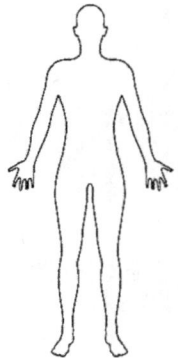

What about your...?

Feeling sick?

Mood   (1)(2)(3)(4)(5)(6)(7)(8)(9)(10)   ☐ Nope!

Energy levels (1)(2)(3)(4)(5)(6)(7)(8)(9)(10)   ☐ Yes...

Mental clarity (1)(2)(3)(4)(5)(6)(7)(8)(9)(10)

☐ Nausea   ☐ Diarrhea   ☐ Vomiting   ☐ Sore throat

☐ Congestion   ☐ Coughing   ☐ Chills   ☐ Fever

Other symptoms: _____

LET'S EXPLORE SOME MORE   #2

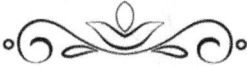

Hours of Sleep ① ② ③ ④ ⑤ ⑥ ⑦ ⑧ ⑨ ⑩ ⊕
Sleep Quality   ① ② ③ ④ ⑤ ⑥ ⑦ ⑧ ⑨ ⑩

WEATHER

☐ Hot   ☐ Mild   ☐ Cold   BM Pressure: _____

☐ Dry   ☐ Humid   ☐ Wet   Allergen Levels: _____

STRESS LEVELS

None	Low	Medium	High	Max	@$#%!

FOOD / MEDICATIONS

FOOD / DRINKS	MEDS / SUPPLEMENTS	TIME	DOSE
	☐ usual daily medication		

EXERCISE / DAILY ACTIVITY

☐ Heck yes, I worked out.

☐ I managed to exercise a bit.

☐ No, I haven't exercised at all.

☐ I did some stuff, and that counts.

DETAILS

NOTES / TRIGGERS / IMPROVEMENTS

_____

_____

_____

WRITE ONE THING YOU'RE GRATEFUL FOR

_____

Date: _____

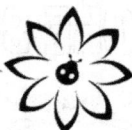

How are you feeling today?

Like death	Terrible	Not good	Meh	Good	Great!	Amazing!

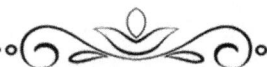

RATE YOUR PAIN LEVEL

① ② ③ ④ ⑤ ⑥ ⑦ ⑧ ⑨ ⑩

Describe your pain / symptoms

	am	pm
	☐	☐
	☐	☐
	☐	☐
	☐	☐
	☐	☐
	☐	☐
	☐	☐
	☐	☐

Where do you feel it?

Front　　　*Back*

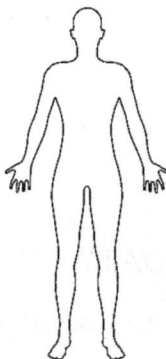

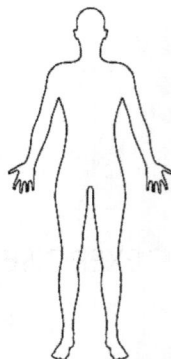

What about your...?

Mood	① ② ③ ④ ⑤ ⑥ ⑦ ⑧ ⑨ ⑩
Energy levels	① ② ③ ④ ⑤ ⑥ ⑦ ⑧ ⑨ ⑩
Mental clarity	① ② ③ ④ ⑤ ⑥ ⑦ ⑧ ⑨ ⑩

Feeling sick?

☐ Nope!

☐ Yes...

☐ Nausea　☐ Diarrhea　☐ Vomiting　☐ Sore throat

☐ Congestion　☐ Coughing　☐ Chills　☐ Fever

Other symptoms: _____

LET'S EXPLORE SOME MORE #3

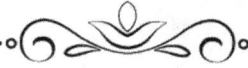

Hours of Sleep (1) (2) (3) (4) (5) (6) (7) (8) (9) (10) (+)

Sleep Quality (1) (2) (3) (4) (5) (6) (7) (8) (9) (10)

WEATHER

☐ Hot   ☐ Mild   ☐ Cold   BM Pressure: _____

☐ Dry   ☐ Humid   ☐ Wet   Allergen Levels: _____

STRESS LEVELS

| None | Low | Medium | High | Max | @$#%! |

FOOD / MEDICATIONS

FOOD / DRINKS	MEDS / SUPPLEMENTS	TIME	DOSE

☐ usual daily medication

EXERCISE / DAILY ACTIVITY

☐ Heck yes, I worked out.

☐ I managed to exercise a bit.

☐ No, I haven't exercised at all.

☐ I did some stuff, and that counts.

DETAILS

NOTES / TRIGGERS / IMPROVEMENTS

WRITE ONE THING YOU'RE GRATEFUL FOR

Date: _____

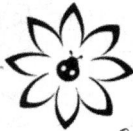

How are you feeling today?

Like death	Terrible	Not good	Meh	Good	Great!	Amazing!

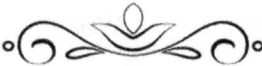

RATE YOUR PAIN LEVEL

(1) (2) (3) (4) (5) (6) (7) (8) (9) (10)

Describe your pain / symptoms   Where do you feel it?

	am	pm
	☐	☐
	☐	☐
	☐	☐
	☐	☐
	☐	☐
	☐	☐
	☐	☐
	☐	☐

Front   Back

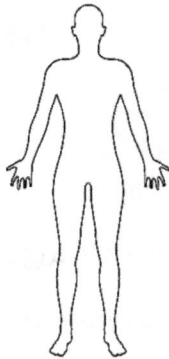

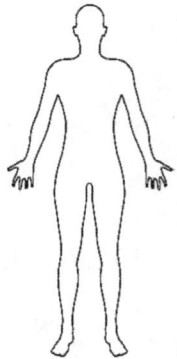

What about your...?   Feeling sick?

Mood (1) (2) (3) (4) (5) (6) (7) (8) (9) (10)   ☐ Nope!

Energy levels (1) (2) (3) (4) (5) (6) (7) (8) (9) (10)   ☐ Yes...

Mental clarity (1) (2) (3) (4) (5) (6) (7) (8) (9) (10)

☐ Nausea   ☐ Diarrhea   ☐ Vomiting   ☐ Sore throat

☐ Congestion   ☐ Coughing   ☐ Chills   ☐ Fever

Other symptoms: _____

LET'S EXPLORE SOME MORE #4

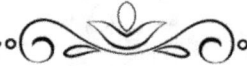

Hours of Sleep (1)(2)(3)(4)(5)(6)(7)(8)(9)(10)(+)

Sleep Quality (1)(2)(3)(4)(5)(6)(7)(8)(9)(10)

WEATHER

☐ Hot   ☐ Mild   ☐ Cold   BM Pressure: _____

☐ Dry   ☐ Humid   ☐ Wet   Allergen Levels: _____

STRESS LEVELS

None	Low	Medium	High	Max	@$#%!

FOOD / MEDICATIONS

FOOD / DRINKS	MEDS / SUPPLEMENTS	TIME	DOSE

☐ usual daily medication

EXERCISE / DAILY ACTIVITY

☐ Heck yes, I worked out.

☐ I managed to exercise a bit.

☐ No, I haven't exercised at all.

☐ I did some stuff, and that counts.

DETAILS

NOTES / TRIGGERS / IMPROVEMENTS

_____

_____

_____

WRITE ONE THING YOU'RE GRATEFUL FOR

_____

Date: _____

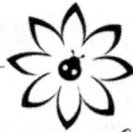

How are you feeling today?

Like death	Terrible	Not good	Meh	Good	Great!	Amazing!

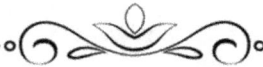

RATE YOUR PAIN LEVEL

(1) (2) (3) (4) (5) (6) (7) (8) (9) (10)

Describe your pain / symptoms

	am	pm
	☐	☐
	☐	☐
	☐	☐
	☐	☐
	☐	☐
	☐	☐
	☐	☐
	☐	☐

Where do you feel it?

Front   *Back*

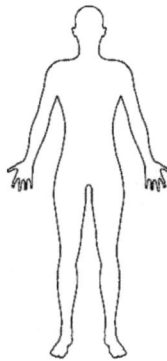

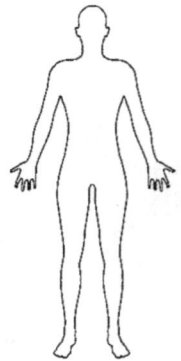

What about your...?

Mood   (1)(2)(3)(4)(5)(6)(7)(8)(9)(10)
Energy levels   (1)(2)(3)(4)(5)(6)(7)(8)(9)(10)
Mental clarity   (1)(2)(3)(4)(5)(6)(7)(8)(9)(10)

Feeling sick?

☐ Nope!
☐ Yes...

☐ Nausea   ☐ Diarrhea   ☐ Vomiting   ☐ Sore throat
☐ Congestion   ☐ Coughing   ☐ Chills   ☐ Fever

Other symptoms: _____

LET'S EXPLORE SOME MORE #5

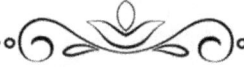

Hours of Sleep ① ② ③ ④ ⑤ ⑥ ⑦ ⑧ ⑨ ⑩ ⊕

Sleep Quality ① ② ③ ④ ⑤ ⑥ ⑦ ⑧ ⑨ ⑩

WEATHER

☐ Hot   ☐ Mild   ☐ Cold   BM Pressure: _____

☐ Dry   ☐ Humid   ☐ Wet   Allergen Levels: _____

STRESS LEVELS

None	Low	Medium	High	Max	@$#%!

FOOD / MEDICATIONS

FOOD / DRINKS	MEDS / SUPPLEMENTS	TIME	DOSE

☐ usual daily medication

EXERCISE / DAILY ACTIVITY

☐ Heck yes, I worked out.

☐ I managed to exercise a bit.

☐ No, I haven't exercised at all.

☐ I did some stuff, and that counts.

DETAILS

NOTES / TRIGGERS / IMPROVEMENTS

_____

_____

_____

WRITE ONE THING YOU'RE GRATEFUL FOR

Date:_____

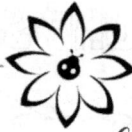

How are you feeling today?

Like death	Terrible	Not good	Meh	Good	Great!	Amazing!

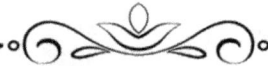

RATE YOUR PAIN LEVEL

① ② ③ ④ ⑤ ⑥ ⑦ ⑧ ⑨ ⑩

Describe your pain / symptoms

Where do you feel it?

	am	pm
	☐	☐
	☐	☐
	☐	☐
	☐	☐
	☐	☐
	☐	☐
	☐	☐
	☐	☐

Front   *Back*

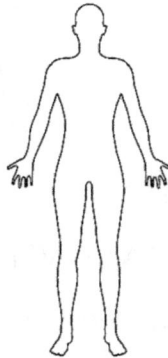

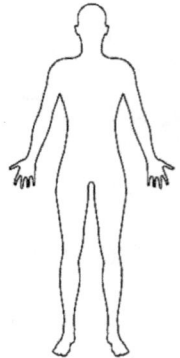

What about your...?

Feeling sick?

Mood	① ② ③ ④ ⑤ ⑥ ⑦ ⑧ ⑨ ⑩	☐ Nope!
Energy levels	① ② ③ ④ ⑤ ⑥ ⑦ ⑧ ⑨ ⑩	☐ Yes...
Mental clarity	① ② ③ ④ ⑤ ⑥ ⑦ ⑧ ⑨ ⑩	

☐ Nausea   ☐ Diarrhea   ☐ Vomiting   ☐ Sore throat

☐ Congestion   ☐ Coughing   ☐ Chills   ☐ Fever

Other symptoms: _____

LET'S EXPLORE SOME MORE #6

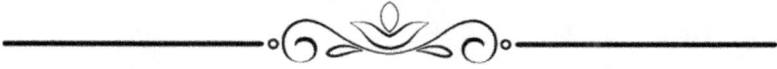

| Hours of Sleep | ① ② ③ ④ ⑤ ⑥ ⑦ ⑧ ⑨ ⑩ ⊕ |
| Sleep Quality | ① ② ③ ④ ⑤ ⑥ ⑦ ⑧ ⑨ ⑩ |

WEATHER

☐ Hot   ☐ Mild   ☐ Cold   BM Pressure: _____

☐ Dry   ☐ Humid   ☐ Wet   Allergen Levels: _____

STRESS LEVELS

| None | Low | Medium | High | Max | @$#%! |

FOOD / MEDICATIONS

FOOD / DRINKS	MEDS / SUPPLEMENTS	TIME	DOSE

☐ usual daily medication

EXERCISE / DAILY ACTIVITY

☐ Heck yes, I worked out.

☐ I managed to exercise a bit.

☐ No, I haven't exercised at all.

☐ I did some stuff, and that counts.

DETAILS

NOTES / TRIGGERS / IMPROVEMENTS

_____

_____

_____

WRITE ONE THING YOU'RE GRATEFUL FOR

Date:_____

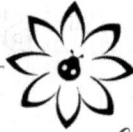

How are you feeling today?

Like death   Terrible   Not good   Meh   Good   Great!   Amazing!

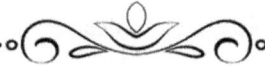

RATE YOUR PAIN LEVEL

(1) (2) (3) (4) (5) (6) (7) (8) (9) (10)

Describe your pain / symptoms   Where do you feel it?

	am	pm
_____	☐	☐
_____	☐	☐
_____	☐	☐
_____	☐	☐
_____	☐	☐
_____	☐	☐
_____	☐	☐
_____	☐	☐

Front   Back

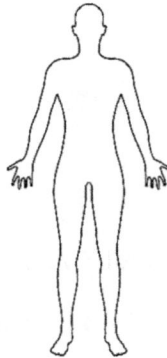

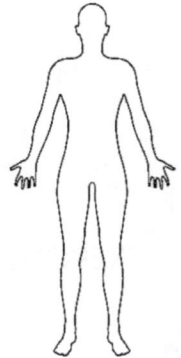

What about your...?   Feeling sick?

Mood	(1)(2)(3)(4)(5)(6)(7)(8)(9)(10)	☐ Nope!
Energy levels	(1)(2)(3)(4)(5)(6)(7)(8)(9)(10)	☐ Yes...
Mental clarity	(1)(2)(3)(4)(5)(6)(7)(8)(9)(10)	

☐ Nausea   ☐ Diarrhea   ☐ Vomiting   ☐ Sore throat

☐ Congestion   ☐ Coughing   ☐ Chills   ☐ Fever

Other symptoms: _____

LET'S EXPLORE SOME MORE #7

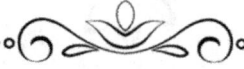

Hours of Sleep (1)(2)(3)(4)(5)(6)(7)(8)(9)(10)(+)

Sleep Quality (1)(2)(3)(4)(5)(6)(7)(8)(9)(10)

WEATHER

☐ Hot ☐ Mild ☐ Cold BM Pressure: _____

☐ Dry ☐ Humid ☐ Wet Allergen Levels: _____

STRESS LEVELS

None	Low	Medium	High	Max	@$#%!

FOOD / MEDICATIONS

FOOD / DRINKS	MEDS / SUPPLEMENTS	TIME	DOSE
	☐ usual daily medication		

EXERCISE / DAILY ACTIVITY

☐ Heck yes, I worked out.

☐ I managed to exercise a bit.

☐ No, I haven't exercised at all.

☐ I did some stuff, and that counts.

DETAILS

NOTES / TRIGGERS / IMPROVEMENTS

_____

_____

_____

WRITE ONE THING YOU'RE GRATEFUL FOR

Date: _____

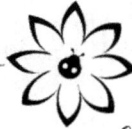

How are you feeling today?

| Like death | Terrible | Not good | Meh | Good | Great! | Amazing! |

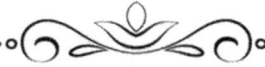

RATE YOUR PAIN LEVEL

(1) (2) (3) (4) (5) (6) (7) (8) (9) (10)

Describe your pain / symptoms

	am	pm
_____	☐	☐
_____	☐	☐
_____	☐	☐
_____	☐	☐
_____	☐	☐
_____	☐	☐
_____	☐	☐
_____	☐	☐

Where do you feel it?

Front   *Back*

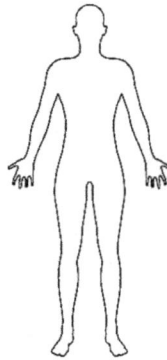

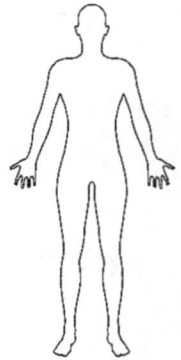

What about your...?

Mood	(1) (2) (3) (4) (5) (6) (7) (8) (9) (10)
Energy levels	(1) (2) (3) (4) (5) (6) (7) (8) (9) (10)
Mental clarity	(1) (2) (3) (4) (5) (6) (7) (8) (9) (10)

Feeling sick?

☐ Nope!

☐ Yes...

☐ Nausea   ☐ Diarrhea   ☐ Vomiting   ☐ Sore throat

☐ Congestion   ☐ Coughing   ☐ Chills   ☐ Fever

Other symptoms: _____

LET'S EXPLORE SOME MORE #8

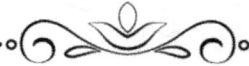

| Hours of Sleep | ① ② ③ ④ ⑤ ⑥ ⑦ ⑧ ⑨ ⑩ ⊕ |
| Sleep Quality | ① ② ③ ④ ⑤ ⑥ ⑦ ⑧ ⑨ ⑩ |

WEATHER

☐ Hot   ☐ Mild   ☐ Cold   BM Pressure: _____

☐ Dry   ☐ Humid   ☐ Wet   Allergen Levels: _____

STRESS LEVELS

| None | Low | Medium | High | Max | @$#%! |

FOOD / MEDICATIONS

FOOD / DRINKS	MEDS / SUPPLEMENTS	TIME	DOSE

☐ usual daily medication

EXERCISE / DAILY ACTIVITY

☐ Heck yes, I worked out.

☐ I managed to exercise a bit.

☐ No, I haven't exercised at all.

☐ I did some stuff, and that counts.

DETAILS

NOTES / TRIGGERS / IMPROVEMENTS

_____

_____

_____

WRITE ONE THING YOU'RE GRATEFUL FOR

_____

Date: _____

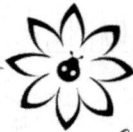

How are you feeling today?

Like death	Terrible	Not good	Meh	Good	Great!	Amazing!

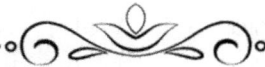

RATE YOUR PAIN LEVEL

(1) (2) (3) (4) (5) (6) (7) (8) (9) (10)

Describe your pain / symptoms

	am	pm
	☐	☐
	☐	☐
	☐	☐
	☐	☐
	☐	☐
	☐	☐
	☐	☐
	☐	☐

Where do you feel it?

Front   *Back*

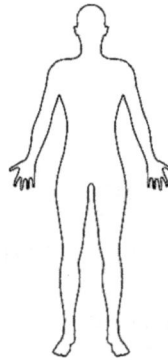

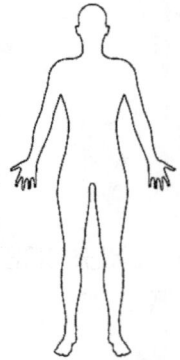

What about your...?

Mood (1) (2) (3) (4) (5) (6) (7) (8) (9) (10)

Energy levels (1) (2) (3) (4) (5) (6) (7) (8) (9) (10)

Mental clarity (1) (2) (3) (4) (5) (6) (7) (8) (9) (10)

Feeling sick?

☐ Nope!

☐ Yes...

☐ Nausea   ☐ Diarrhea   ☐ Vomiting   ☐ Sore throat

☐ Congestion   ☐ Coughing   ☐ Chills   ☐ Fever

Other symptoms: _____

LET'S EXPLORE SOME MORE #9

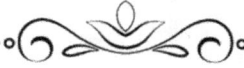

Hours of Sleep ① ② ③ ④ ⑤ ⑥ ⑦ ⑧ ⑨ ⑩ ⊕

Sleep Quality ① ② ③ ④ ⑤ ⑥ ⑦ ⑧ ⑨ ⑩

WEATHER

☐ Hot ☐ Mild ☐ Cold BM Pressure: _____

☐ Dry ☐ Humid ☐ Wet Allergen Levels: _____

STRESS LEVELS

| None | Low | Medium | High | Max | @$#%! |

FOOD / MEDICATIONS

FOOD / DRINKS	MEDS / SUPPLEMENTS	TIME	DOSE

☐ usual daily medication

EXERCISE / DAILY ACTIVITY

☐ Heck yes, I worked out.

☐ I managed to exercise a bit.

☐ No, I haven't exercised at all.

☐ I did some stuff, and that counts.

DETAILS

NOTES / TRIGGERS / IMPROVEMENTS

WRITE ONE THING YOU'RE GRATEFUL FOR

Date: _____

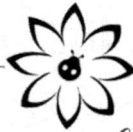

How are you feeling today?

| Like death | Terrible | Not good | Meh | Good | Great! | Amazing! |

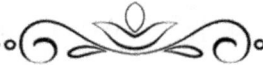

RATE YOUR PAIN LEVEL

① ② ③ ④ ⑤ ⑥ ⑦ ⑧ ⑨ ⑩

Describe your pain / symptoms

	am	pm
_____	☐	☐
_____	☐	☐
_____	☐	☐
_____	☐	☐
_____	☐	☐
_____	☐	☐
_____	☐	☐
_____	☐	☐

Where do you feel it?

Front   Back

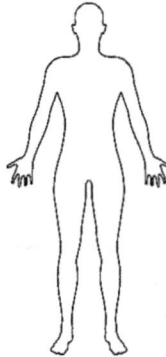

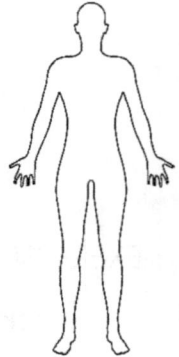

What about your...?

Mood	① ② ③ ④ ⑤ ⑥ ⑦ ⑧ ⑨ ⑩
Energy levels	① ② ③ ④ ⑤ ⑥ ⑦ ⑧ ⑨ ⑩
Mental clarity	① ② ③ ④ ⑤ ⑥ ⑦ ⑧ ⑨ ⑩

Feeling sick?

☐ Nope!
☐ Yes...

☐ Nausea   ☐ Diarrhea   ☐ Vomiting   ☐ Sore throat
☐ Congestion   ☐ Coughing   ☐ Chills   ☐ Fever

Other symptoms: _____

LET'S EXPLORE SOME MORE #10

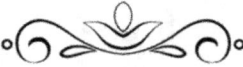

Hours of Sleep ① ② ③ ④ ⑤ ⑥ ⑦ ⑧ ⑨ ⑩ ⊕

Sleep Quality ① ② ③ ④ ⑤ ⑥ ⑦ ⑧ ⑨ ⑩

WEATHER

☐ Hot   ☐ Mild   ☐ Cold   BM Pressure: _____

☐ Dry   ☐ Humid   ☐ Wet   Allergen Levels: _____

STRESS LEVELS

None	Low	Medium	High	Max	@$#%!

FOOD / MEDICATIONS

FOOD / DRINKS	MEDS / SUPPLEMENTS	TIME	DOSE

☐ usual daily medication

EXERCISE / DAILY ACTIVITY

☐ Heck yes, I worked out.

☐ I managed to exercise a bit.

☐ No, I haven't exercised at all.

☐ I did some stuff, and that counts.

DETAILS

NOTES / TRIGGERS / IMPROVEMENTS

_____

_____

_____

WRITE ONE THING YOU'RE GRATEFUL FOR

_____

Date: _____

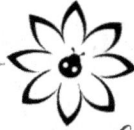

How are you feeling today?

| Like death | Terrible | Not good | Meh | Good | Great! | Amazing! |

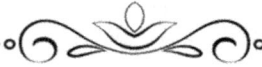

RATE YOUR PAIN LEVEL

(1) (2) (3) (4) (5) (6) (7) (8) (9) (10)

Describe your pain / symptoms

Where do you feel it?

am	pm
☐	☐
☐	☐
☐	☐
☐	☐
☐	☐
☐	☐
☐	☐
☐	☐

Front   Back

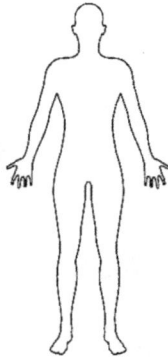

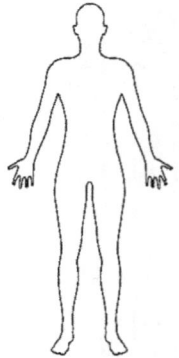

What about your...?

Feeling sick?

Mood	1 2 3 4 5 6 7 8 9 10	☐ Nope!
Energy levels	1 2 3 4 5 6 7 8 9 10	☐ Yes...
Mental clarity	1 2 3 4 5 6 7 8 9 10	

☐ Nausea   ☐ Diarrhea   ☐ Vomiting   ☐ Sore throat

☐ Congestion   ☐ Coughing   ☐ Chills   ☐ Fever

Other symptoms: _____

LET'S EXPLORE SOME MORE #11

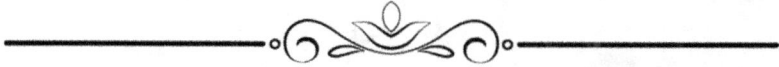

Hours of Sleep ① ② ③ ④ ⑤ ⑥ ⑦ ⑧ ⑨ ⑩ ⊕
Sleep Quality ① ② ③ ④ ⑤ ⑥ ⑦ ⑧ ⑨ ⑩

WEATHER

☐ Hot ☐ Mild ☐ Cold BM Pressure: _____

☐ Dry ☐ Humid ☐ Wet Allergen Levels: _____

STRESS LEVELS

None	Low	Medium	High	Max	@$#%!

FOOD / MEDICATIONS

FOOD / DRINKS	MEDS / SUPPLEMENTS	TIME	DOSE

☐ usual daily medication

EXERCISE / DAILY ACTIVITY

☐ Heck yes, I worked out.

☐ I managed to exercise a bit.

☐ No, I haven't exercised at all.

☐ I did some stuff, and that counts.

DETAILS

NOTES / TRIGGERS / IMPROVEMENTS

_____

_____

_____

WRITE ONE THING YOU'RE GRATEFUL FOR

_____

Date: _____

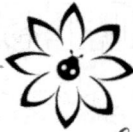

How are you feeling today?

😵	😖	😠	🙂	😊	😁	😍
Like death	Terrible	Not good	Meh	Good	Great!	Amazing!

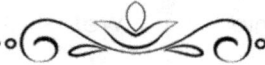

RATE YOUR PAIN LEVEL

① ② ③ ④ ⑤ ⑥ ⑦ ⑧ ⑨ ⑩

Describe your pain / symptoms

	am	pm
_____	☐	☐
_____	☐	☐
_____	☐	☐
_____	☐	☐
_____	☐	☐
_____	☐	☐
_____	☐	☐
_____	☐	☐

Where do you feel it?

Front   *Back*

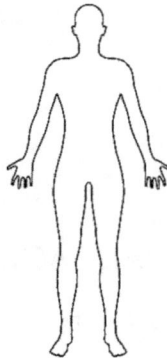 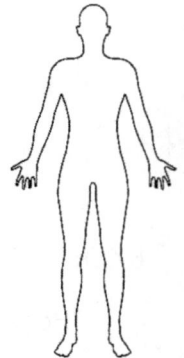

What about your...?

		Feeling sick?
Mood	①②③④⑤⑥⑦⑧⑨⑩	☐ Nope!
Energy levels	①②③④⑤⑥⑦⑧⑨⑩	☐ Yes...
Mental clarity	①②③④⑤⑥⑦⑧⑨⑩	

☐ Nausea   ☐ Diarrhea   ☐ Vomiting   ☐ Sore throat

☐ Congestion   ☐ Coughing   ☐ Chills   ☐ Fever

Other symptoms: _____

LET'S EXPLORE SOME MORE #12

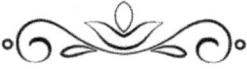

Hours of Sleep (1) (2) (3) (4) (5) (6) (7) (8) (9) (10) (+)

Sleep Quality (1) (2) (3) (4) (5) (6) (7) (8) (9) (10)

WEATHER

☐ Hot ☐ Mild ☐ Cold BM Pressure: _____

☐ Dry ☐ Humid ☐ Wet Allergen Levels: _____

STRESS LEVELS

| None | Low | Medium | High | Max | @$#%! |

FOOD / MEDICATIONS

FOOD / DRINKS	MEDS / SUPPLEMENTS	TIME	DOSE

☐ usual daily medication

EXERCISE / DAILY ACTIVITY

DETAILS

☐ Heck yes, I worked out.

☐ I managed to exercise a bit.

☐ No, I haven't exercised at all.

☐ I did some stuff, and that counts.

NOTES / TRIGGERS / IMPROVEMENTS

WRITE ONE THING YOU'RE GRATEFUL FOR

Date: _____

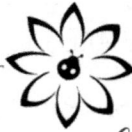

How are you feeling today?

Like death	Terrible	Not good	Meh	Good	Great!	Amazing!

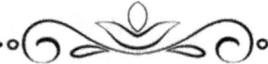

RATE YOUR PAIN LEVEL

① ② ③ ④ ⑤ ⑥ ⑦ ⑧ ⑨ ⑩

Describe your pain / symptoms

Where do you feel it?

	am	pm
_____	☐	☐
_____	☐	☐
_____	☐	☐
_____	☐	☐
_____	☐	☐
_____	☐	☐
_____	☐	☐
_____	☐	☐

Front   *Back*

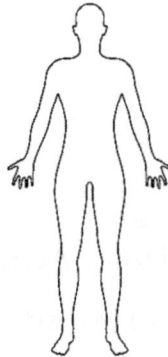

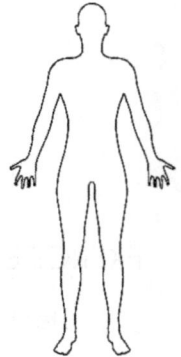

What about your...?   Feeling sick?

Mood	① ② ③ ④ ⑤ ⑥ ⑦ ⑧ ⑨ ⑩	☐ Nope!
Energy levels	① ② ③ ④ ⑤ ⑥ ⑦ ⑧ ⑨ ⑩	☐ Yes...
Mental clarity	① ② ③ ④ ⑤ ⑥ ⑦ ⑧ ⑨ ⑩	

☐ Nausea   ☐ Diarrhea   ☐ Vomiting   ☐ Sore throat

☐ Congestion   ☐ Coughing   ☐ Chills   ☐ Fever

Other symptoms: _____

LET'S EXPLORE SOME MORE #13

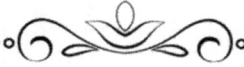

| Hours of Sleep | ① ② ③ ④ ⑤ ⑥ ⑦ ⑧ ⑨ ⑩ ⊕ |
| Sleep Quality | ① ② ③ ④ ⑤ ⑥ ⑦ ⑧ ⑨ ⑩ |

WEATHER

☐ Hot ☐ Mild ☐ Cold   BM Pressure: _____

☐ Dry ☐ Humid ☐ Wet   Allergen Levels: _____

STRESS LEVELS

| None | Low | Medium | High | Max | @$#%! |

FOOD / MEDICATIONS

FOOD / DRINKS	MEDS / SUPPLEMENTS	TIME	DOSE

☐ usual daily medication

EXERCISE / DAILY ACTIVITY

☐ Heck yes, I worked out.

☐ I managed to exercise a bit.

☐ No, I haven't exercised at all.

☐ I did some stuff, and that counts.

DETAILS

NOTES / TRIGGERS / IMPROVEMENTS

WRITE ONE THING YOU'RE GRATEFUL FOR

Date: _____

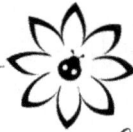

How are you feeling today?

😣	😖	😠	🙂	😊	😁	😍
Like death	Terrible	Not good	Meh	Good	Great!	Amazing!

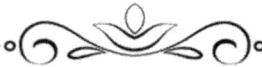

RATE YOUR PAIN LEVEL

① ② ③ ④ ⑤ ⑥ ⑦ ⑧ ⑨ ⑩

Describe your pain / symptoms			Where do you feel it?

	am	pm
	☐	☐
	☐	☐
	☐	☐
	☐	☐
	☐	☐
	☐	☐
	☐	☐
	☐	☐

Front   *Back*

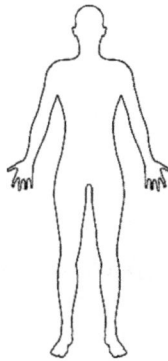

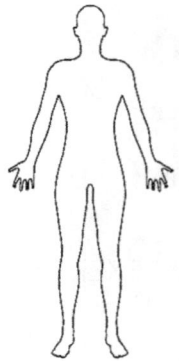

What about your...?   Feeling sick?

Mood	① ② ③ ④ ⑤ ⑥ ⑦ ⑧ ⑨ ⑩	☐ Nope!
Energy levels	① ② ③ ④ ⑤ ⑥ ⑦ ⑧ ⑨ ⑩	☐ Yes...
Mental clarity	① ② ③ ④ ⑤ ⑥ ⑦ ⑧ ⑨ ⑩	

☐ Nausea   ☐ Diarrhea   ☐ Vomiting   ☐ Sore throat

☐ Congestion   ☐ Coughing   ☐ Chills   ☐ Fever

Other symptoms: _____

LET'S EXPLORE SOME MORE #14

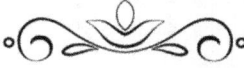

| Hours of Sleep | ① ② ③ ④ ⑤ ⑥ ⑦ ⑧ ⑨ ⑩ ⊕ |
| Sleep Quality | ① ② ③ ④ ⑤ ⑥ ⑦ ⑧ ⑨ ⑩ |

WEATHER

☐ Hot ☐ Mild ☐ Cold BM Pressure: _____

☐ Dry ☐ Humid ☐ Wet Allergen Levels: _____

STRESS LEVELS

| None | Low | Medium | High | Max | @$#%! |

FOOD / MEDICATIONS

FOOD / DRINKS	MEDS / SUPPLEMENTS	TIME	DOSE

☐ usual daily medication

EXERCISE / DAILY ACTIVITY

☐ Heck yes, I worked out.

☐ I managed to exercise a bit.

☐ No, I haven't exercised at all.

☐ I did some stuff, and that counts.

DETAILS

NOTES / TRIGGERS / IMPROVEMENTS

_____

_____

_____

WRITE ONE THING YOU'RE GRATEFUL FOR

_____

Date: _____

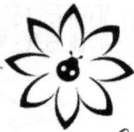

How are you feeling today?

😵	😣	😠	🙂	😊	😁	😍
Like death	Terrible	Not good	Meh	Good	Great!	Amazing!

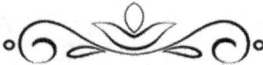

RATE YOUR PAIN LEVEL

① ② ③ ④ ⑤ ⑥ ⑦ ⑧ ⑨ ⑩

Describe your pain / symptoms   Where do you feel it?

	am	pm
	☐	☐
	☐	☐
	☐	☐
	☐	☐
	☐	☐
	☐	☐
	☐	☐
	☐	☐

Front   *Back*

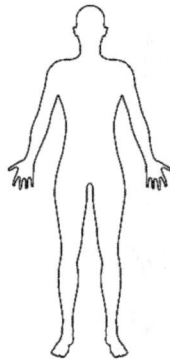 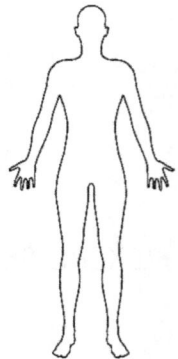

What about your...?   Feeling sick?

Mood	① ② ③ ④ ⑤ ⑥ ⑦ ⑧ ⑨ ⑩	☐ Nope!
Energy levels	① ② ③ ④ ⑤ ⑥ ⑦ ⑧ ⑨ ⑩	☐ Yes...
Mental clarity	① ② ③ ④ ⑤ ⑥ ⑦ ⑧ ⑨ ⑩	

☐ Nausea   ☐ Diarrhea   ☐ Vomiting   ☐ Sore throat

☐ Congestion ☐ Coughing   ☐ Chills   ☐ Fever

Other symptoms: _____

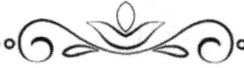

LET'S EXPLORE SOME MORE #15

Hours of Sleep ① ② ③ ④ ⑤ ⑥ ⑦ ⑧ ⑨ ⑩ ⊕

Sleep Quality ① ② ③ ④ ⑤ ⑥ ⑦ ⑧ ⑨ ⑩

WEATHER

☐ Hot   ☐ Mild   ☐ Cold   BM Pressure: _____

☐ Dry   ☐ Humid   ☐ Wet   Allergen Levels: _____

STRESS LEVELS

None	Low	Medium	High	Max	@$#%!

FOOD / MEDICATIONS

FOOD / DRINKS	MEDS / SUPPLEMENTS	TIME	DOSE

☐ usual daily medication

EXERCISE / DAILY ACTIVITY

☐ Heck yes, I worked out.

☐ I managed to exercise a bit.

☐ No, I haven't exercised at all.

☐ I did some stuff, and that counts.

DETAILS

NOTES / TRIGGERS / IMPROVEMENTS

_____

_____

_____

WRITE ONE THING YOU'RE GRATEFUL FOR

_____

Date: _____

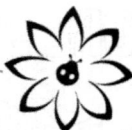

How are you feeling today?

Like death	Terrible	Not good	Meh	Good	Great!	Amazing!

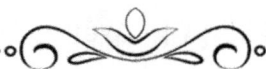

RATE YOUR PAIN LEVEL

① ② ③ ④ ⑤ ⑥ ⑦ ⑧ ⑨ ⑩

Describe your pain / symptoms

Where do you feel it?

	am	pm
_____	☐	☐
_____	☐	☐
_____	☐	☐
_____	☐	☐
_____	☐	☐
_____	☐	☐
_____	☐	☐
_____	☐	☐

Front   *Back*

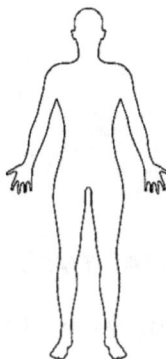

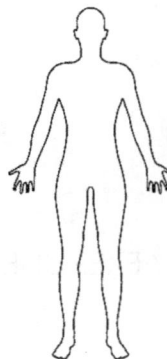

What about your...?

Feeling sick?

Mood   ① ② ③ ④ ⑤ ⑥ ⑦ ⑧ ⑨ ⑩   ☐ Nope!
Energy levels   ① ② ③ ④ ⑤ ⑥ ⑦ ⑧ ⑨ ⑩   ☐ Yes...
Mental clarity ① ② ③ ④ ⑤ ⑥ ⑦ ⑧ ⑨ ⑩

☐ Nausea   ☐ Diarrhea   ☐ Vomiting   ☐ Sore throat
☐ Congestion   ☐ Coughing   ☐ Chills   ☐ Fever

Other symptoms: _____

LET'S EXPLORE SOME MORE #16

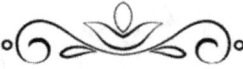

Hours of Sleep (1) (2) (3) (4) (5) (6) (7) (8) (9) (10) (+)

Sleep Quality (1) (2) (3) (4) (5) (6) (7) (8) (9) (10)

WEATHER

☐ Hot   ☐ Mild   ☐ Cold   BM Pressure: _____

☐ Dry   ☐ Humid   ☐ Wet   Allergen Levels: _____

STRESS LEVELS

None	Low	Medium	High	Max	@$#%!

FOOD / MEDICATIONS

FOOD / DRINKS	MEDS / SUPPLEMENTS	TIME	DOSE

☐ usual daily medication

EXERCISE / DAILY ACTIVITY

☐ Heck yes, I worked out.

☐ I managed to exercise a bit.

☐ No, I haven't exercised at all.

☐ I did some stuff, and that counts.

DETAILS

NOTES / TRIGGERS / IMPROVEMENTS

_____

_____

_____

WRITE ONE THING YOU'RE GRATEFUL FOR

Date: _____

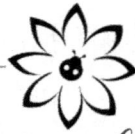

How are you feeling today?

Like death	Terrible	Not good	Meh	Good	Great!	Amazing!

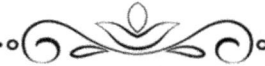

RATE YOUR PAIN LEVEL

(1) (2) (3) (4) (5) (6) (7) (8) (9) (10)

Describe your pain / symptoms

	am	pm
	☐	☐
	☐	☐
	☐	☐
	☐	☐
	☐	☐
	☐	☐
	☐	☐
	☐	☐

Where do you feel it?

Front   Back

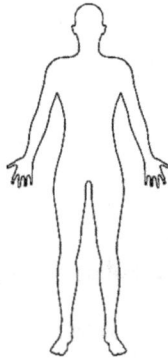

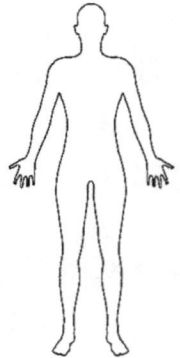

What about your...?

Mood   (1) (2) (3) (4) (5) (6) (7) (8) (9) (10)
Energy levels (1) (2) (3) (4) (5) (6) (7) (8) (9) (10)
Mental clarity (1) (2) (3) (4) (5) (6) (7) (8) (9) (10)

Feeling sick?

☐ Nope!
☐ Yes...

☐ Nausea   ☐ Diarrhea   ☐ Vomiting   ☐ Sore throat
☐ Congestion ☐ Coughing   ☐ Chills   ☐ Fever

Other symptoms: _____

LET'S EXPLORE SOME MORE #17

Hours of Sleep ① ② ③ ④ ⑤ ⑥ ⑦ ⑧ ⑨ ⑩ ⊕

Sleep Quality ① ② ③ ④ ⑤ ⑥ ⑦ ⑧ ⑨ ⑩

WEATHER

☐ Hot   ☐ Mild   ☐ Cold   BM Pressure: _____

☐ Dry   ☐ Humid   ☐ Wet   Allergen Levels: _____

STRESS LEVELS

| None | Low | Medium | High | Max | @$#%! |

FOOD / MEDICATIONS

FOOD / DRINKS	MEDS / SUPPLEMENTS	TIME	DOSE

☐ usual daily medication

EXERCISE / DAILY ACTIVITY

☐ Heck yes, I worked out.

☐ I managed to exercise a bit.

☐ No, I haven't exercised at all.

☐ I did some stuff, and that counts.

DETAILS

NOTES / TRIGGERS / IMPROVEMENTS

_____

_____

_____

WRITE ONE THING YOU'RE GRATEFUL FOR

_____

Date: _____

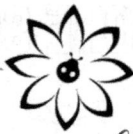

How are you feeling today?

😵 Like death   😣 Terrible   😠 Not good   🙂 Meh   😊 Good   😁 Great!   😍 Amazing!

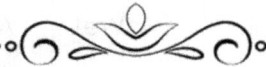

RATE YOUR PAIN LEVEL

① ② ③ ④ ⑤ ⑥ ⑦ ⑧ ⑨ ⑩

Describe your pain / symptoms

	am	pm
	☐	☐
	☐	☐
	☐	☐
	☐	☐
	☐	☐
	☐	☐
	☐	☐
	☐	☐

Where do you feel it?

Front   *Back*

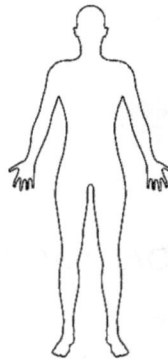 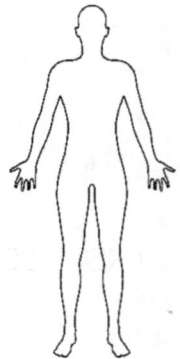

What about your...?

Mood	① ② ③ ④ ⑤ ⑥ ⑦ ⑧ ⑨ ⑩
Energy levels	① ② ③ ④ ⑤ ⑥ ⑦ ⑧ ⑨ ⑩
Mental clarity	① ② ③ ④ ⑤ ⑥ ⑦ ⑧ ⑨ ⑩

Feeling sick?

☐ Nope!
☐ Yes...

☐ Nausea   ☐ Diarrhea   ☐ Vomiting   ☐ Sore throat
☐ Congestion ☐ Coughing   ☐ Chills   ☐ Fever

Other symptoms: _____

LET'S EXPLORE SOME MORE #18

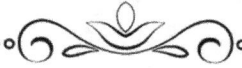

Hours of Sleep ① ② ③ ④ ⑤ ⑥ ⑦ ⑧ ⑨ ⑩ ⊕
Sleep Quality ① ② ③ ④ ⑤ ⑥ ⑦ ⑧ ⑨ ⑩

WEATHER

☐ Hot ☐ Mild ☐ Cold BM Pressure: _____

☐ Dry ☐ Humid ☐ Wet Allergen Levels: _____

STRESS LEVELS

None	Low	Medium	High	Max	@$#%!

FOOD / MEDICATIONS

FOOD / DRINKS	MEDS / SUPPLEMENTS	TIME	DOSE

☐ usual daily medication

EXERCISE / DAILY ACTIVITY

☐ Heck yes, I worked out.

☐ I managed to exercise a bit.

☐ No, I haven't exercised at all.

☐ I did some stuff, and that counts.

DETAILS

NOTES / TRIGGERS / IMPROVEMENTS

WRITE ONE THING YOU'RE GRATEFUL FOR

Date: _____

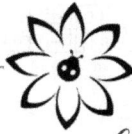

How are you feeling today?

Like death	Terrible	Not good	Meh	Good	Great!	Amazing!

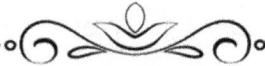

RATE YOUR PAIN LEVEL

(1) (2) (3) (4) (5) (6) (7) (8) (9) (10)

Describe your pain / symptoms

	am	pm
	☐	☐
	☐	☐
	☐	☐
	☐	☐
	☐	☐
	☐	☐
	☐	☐
	☐	☐

Where do you feel it?

Front   *Back*

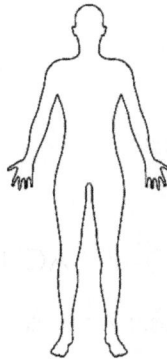

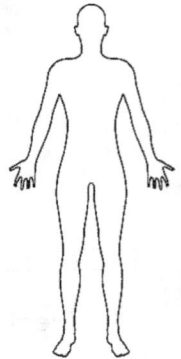

What about your...?

Mood	(1) (2) (3) (4) (5) (6) (7) (8) (9) (10)
Energy levels	(1) (2) (3) (4) (5) (6) (7) (8) (9) (10)
Mental clarity	(1) (2) (3) (4) (5) (6) (7) (8) (9) (10)

Feeling sick?

☐ Nope!

☐ Yes...

☐ Nausea   ☐ Diarrhea   ☐ Vomiting   ☐ Sore throat

☐ Congestion   ☐ Coughing   ☐ Chills   ☐ Fever

Other symptoms: _____

LET'S EXPLORE SOME MORE #19

Hours of Sleep ① ② ③ ④ ⑤ ⑥ ⑦ ⑧ ⑨ ⑩ ⊕

Sleep Quality ① ② ③ ④ ⑤ ⑥ ⑦ ⑧ ⑨ ⑩

WEATHER

☐ Hot   ☐ Mild   ☐ Cold   BM Pressure: _____

☐ Dry   ☐ Humid ☐ Wet   Allergen Levels: _____

STRESS LEVELS

None	Low	Medium	High	Max	@$#%!

FOOD / MEDICATIONS

FOOD / DRINKS	MEDS / SUPPLEMENTS	TIME	DOSE

☐ usual daily medication

EXERCISE / DAILY ACTIVITY

☐ Heck yes, I worked out.

☐ I managed to exercise a bit.

☐ No, I haven't exercised at all.

☐ I did some stuff, and that counts.

DETAILS

NOTES / TRIGGERS / IMPROVEMENTS

_____

_____

_____

WRITE ONE THING YOU'RE GRATEFUL FOR

_____

Date:_____

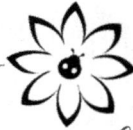

How are you feeling today?

Like death	Terrible	Not good	Meh	Good	Great!	Amazing!

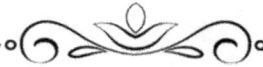

RATE YOUR PAIN LEVEL

① ② ③ ④ ⑤ ⑥ ⑦ ⑧ ⑨ ⑩

Describe your pain / symptoms

Where do you feel it?

am	pm
☐	☐
☐	☐
☐	☐
☐	☐
☐	☐
☐	☐
☐	☐
☐	☐

Front   *Back*

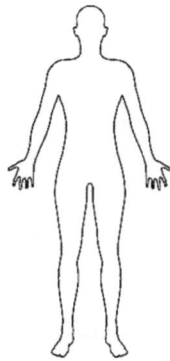

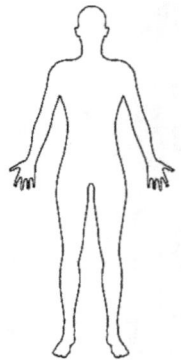

What about your...?

Feeling sick?

Mood	① ② ③ ④ ⑤ ⑥ ⑦ ⑧ ⑨ ⑩	☐ Nope!
Energy levels	① ② ③ ④ ⑤ ⑥ ⑦ ⑧ ⑨ ⑩	☐ Yes...
Mental clarity	① ② ③ ④ ⑤ ⑥ ⑦ ⑧ ⑨ ⑩	

☐ Nausea   ☐ Diarrhea   ☐ Vomiting   ☐ Sore throat

☐ Congestion   ☐ Coughing   ☐ Chills   ☐ Fever

Other symptoms: _____

LET'S EXPLORE SOME MORE #20

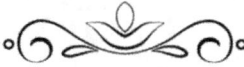

Hours of Sleep (1) (2) (3) (4) (5) (6) (7) (8) (9) (10) (+)

Sleep Quality (1) (2) (3) (4) (5) (6) (7) (8) (9) (10)

WEATHER

☐ Hot   ☐ Mild   ☐ Cold   BM Pressure: _____

☐ Dry   ☐ Humid   ☐ Wet   Allergen Levels: _____

STRESS LEVELS

None	Low	Medium	High	Max	@$#%!

FOOD / MEDICATIONS

FOOD / DRINKS	MEDS / SUPPLEMENTS	TIME	DOSE

☐ usual daily medication

EXERCISE / DAILY ACTIVITY

☐ Heck yes, I worked out.

☐ I managed to exercise a bit.

☐ No, I haven't exercised at all.

☐ I did some stuff, and that counts.

DETAILS

NOTES / TRIGGERS / IMPROVEMENTS

_____

_____

_____

WRITE ONE THING YOU'RE GRATEFUL FOR

_____

Date: _____

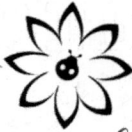

How are you feeling today?

Like death	Terrible	Not good	Meh	Good	Great!	Amazing!

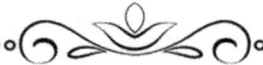

RATE YOUR PAIN LEVEL

① ② ③ ④ ⑤ ⑥ ⑦ ⑧ ⑨ ⑩

Describe your pain / symptoms

Where do you feel it?

	am	pm
_____	☐	☐
_____	☐	☐
_____	☐	☐
_____	☐	☐
_____	☐	☐
_____	☐	☐
_____	☐	☐
_____	☐	☐

Front   *Back*

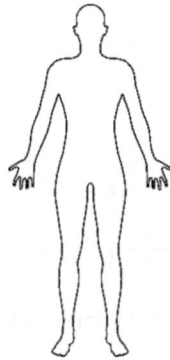 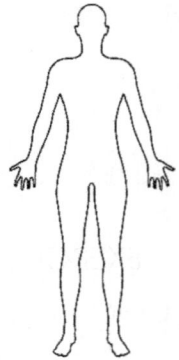

What about your...?

Feeling sick?

Mood ① ② ③ ④ ⑤ ⑥ ⑦ ⑧ ⑨ ⑩   ☐ Nope!

Energy levels ① ② ③ ④ ⑤ ⑥ ⑦ ⑧ ⑨ ⑩   ☐ Yes...

Mental clarity ① ② ③ ④ ⑤ ⑥ ⑦ ⑧ ⑨ ⑩

☐ Nausea   ☐ Diarrhea   ☐ Vomiting   ☐ Sore throat

☐ Congestion ☐ Coughing   ☐ Chills   ☐ Fever

Other symptoms: _____

LET'S EXPLORE SOME MORE #21

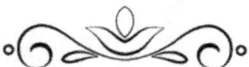

Hours of Sleep (1)(2)(3)(4)(5)(6)(7)(8)(9)(10)(+)

Sleep Quality (1)(2)(3)(4)(5)(6)(7)(8)(9)(10)

WEATHER

☐ Hot   ☐ Mild   ☐ Cold   BM Pressure: _____

☐ Dry   ☐ Humid   ☐ Wet   Allergen Levels: _____

STRESS LEVELS

None	Low	Medium	High	Max	@$#%!

FOOD / MEDICATIONS

FOOD / DRINKS	MEDS / SUPPLEMENTS	TIME	DOSE

☐ usual daily medication

EXERCISE / DAILY ACTIVITY

☐ Heck yes, I worked out.

☐ I managed to exercise a bit.

☐ No, I haven't exercised at all.

☐ I did some stuff, and that counts.

DETAILS

NOTES / TRIGGERS / IMPROVEMENTS

_____

_____

_____

WRITE ONE THING YOU'RE GRATEFUL FOR

Date:_____

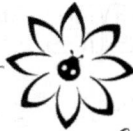

How are you feeling today?

| Like death | Terrible | Not good | Meh | Good | Great! | Amazing! |

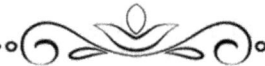

RATE YOUR PAIN LEVEL

(1) (2) (3) (4) (5) (6) (7) (8) (9) (10)

Describe your pain / symptoms

	am	pm
	☐	☐
	☐	☐
	☐	☐
	☐	☐
	☐	☐
	☐	☐
	☐	☐
	☐	☐

Where do you feel it?

Front   *Back*

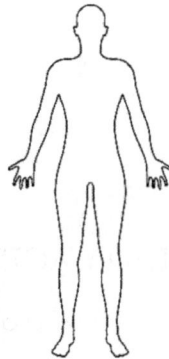

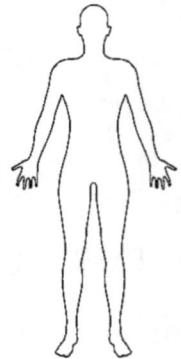

What about your...?

Mood   (1) (2) (3) (4) (5) (6) (7) (8) (9) (10)
Energy levels   (1) (2) (3) (4) (5) (6) (7) (8) (9) (10)
Mental clarity   (1) (2) (3) (4) (5) (6) (7) (8) (9) (10)

Feeling sick?

☐ Nope!
☐ Yes...

☐ Nausea   ☐ Diarrhea   ☐ Vomiting   ☐ Sore throat
☐ Congestion ☐ Coughing   ☐ Chills   ☐ Fever

Other symptoms:

LET'S EXPLORE SOME MORE #22

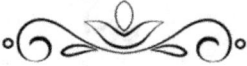

Hours of Sleep ① ② ③ ④ ⑤ ⑥ ⑦ ⑧ ⑨ ⑩ ⊕

Sleep Quality ① ② ③ ④ ⑤ ⑥ ⑦ ⑧ ⑨ ⑩

WEATHER

☐ Hot ☐ Mild ☐ Cold BM Pressure: _____

☐ Dry ☐ Humid ☐ Wet Allergen Levels: _____

STRESS LEVELS

None	Low	Medium	High	Max	@$#%!

FOOD / MEDICATIONS

FOOD / DRINKS	MEDS / SUPPLEMENTS	TIME	DOSE

☐ usual daily medication

EXERCISE / DAILY ACTIVITY

☐ Heck yes, I worked out.

☐ I managed to exercise a bit.

☐ No, I haven't exercised at all.

☐ I did some stuff, and that counts.

DETAILS

NOTES / TRIGGERS / IMPROVEMENTS

_____

_____

WRITE ONE THING YOU'RE GRATEFUL FOR

Date: _____

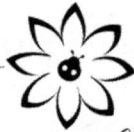

How are you feeling today?

Like death	Terrible	Not good	Meh	Good	Great!	Amazing!

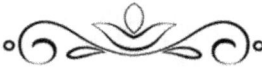

RATE YOUR PAIN LEVEL

(1) (2) (3) (4) (5) (6) (7) (8) (9) (10)

Describe your pain / symptoms   Where do you feel it?

	am	pm
	☐	☐
	☐	☐
	☐	☐
	☐	☐
	☐	☐
	☐	☐
	☐	☐
	☐	☐

Front   *Back*

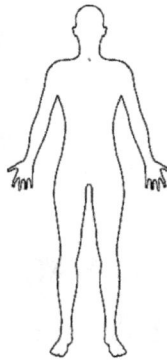

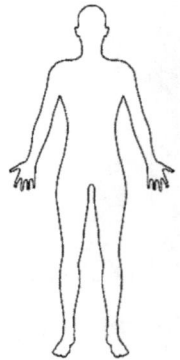

What about your...?   Feeling sick?

Mood	(1) (2) (3) (4) (5) (6) (7) (8) (9) (10)	☐ Nope!
Energy levels	(1) (2) (3) (4) (5) (6) (7) (8) (9) (10)	☐ Yes...
Mental clarity	(1) (2) (3) (4) (5) (6) (7) (8) (9) (10)	

☐ Nausea	☐ Diarrhea	☐ Vomiting	☐ Sore throat
☐ Congestion	☐ Coughing	☐ Chills	☐ Fever

Other symptoms: _____

LET'S EXPLORE SOME MORE #23

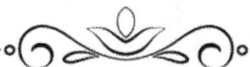

Hours of Sleep ① ② ③ ④ ⑤ ⑥ ⑦ ⑧ ⑨ ⑩ ⊕

Sleep Quality ① ② ③ ④ ⑤ ⑥ ⑦ ⑧ ⑨ ⑩

WEATHER

☐ Hot   ☐ Mild   ☐ Cold   BM Pressure: _____

☐ Dry   ☐ Humid   ☐ Wet   Allergen Levels: _____

STRESS LEVELS

None	Low	Medium	High	Max	@$#%!

FOOD / MEDICATIONS

FOOD / DRINKS	MEDS / SUPPLEMENTS	TIME	DOSE

☐ usual daily medication

EXERCISE / DAILY ACTIVITY

☐ Heck yes, I worked out.

☐ I managed to exercise a bit.

☐ No, I haven't exercised at all.

☐ I did some stuff, and that counts.

DETAILS

NOTES / TRIGGERS / IMPROVEMENTS

_____

_____

_____

WRITE ONE THING YOU'RE GRATEFUL FOR

_____

Date:_____

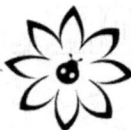

How are you feeling today?

😵	😖	☹️	🙂	😊	😁	😍
Like death	Terrible	Not good	Meh	Good	Great!	Amazing!

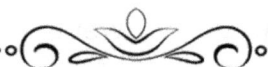

RATE YOUR PAIN LEVEL

① ② ③ ④ ⑤ ⑥ ⑦ ⑧ ⑨ ⑩

Describe your pain / symptoms   Where do you feel it?

	am	pm
_____	☐	☐
_____	☐	☐
_____	☐	☐
_____	☐	☐
_____	☐	☐
_____	☐	☐
_____	☐	☐
_____	☐	☐

Front

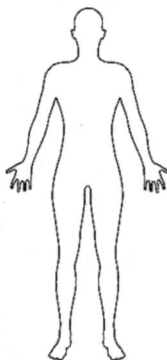

Back

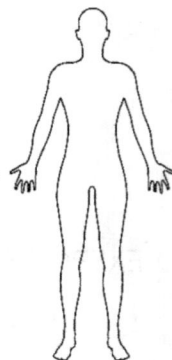

What about your...?   Feeling sick?

Mood   ① ② ③ ④ ⑤ ⑥ ⑦ ⑧ ⑨ ⑩   ☐ Nope!

Energy levels   ① ② ③ ④ ⑤ ⑥ ⑦ ⑧ ⑨ ⑩   ☐ Yes...

Mental clarity ① ② ③ ④ ⑤ ⑥ ⑦ ⑧ ⑨ ⑩

☐ Nausea   ☐ Diarrhea   ☐ Vomiting   ☐ Sore throat

☐ Congestion   ☐ Coughing   ☐ Chills   ☐ Fever

Other symptoms: _____

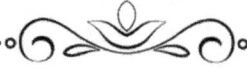

| Hours of Sleep | ① ② ③ ④ ⑤ ⑥ ⑦ ⑧ ⑨ ⑩ ⊕ |
| Sleep Quality | ① ② ③ ④ ⑤ ⑥ ⑦ ⑧ ⑨ ⑩ |

WEATHER

☐ Hot   ☐ Mild   ☐ Cold   BM Pressure: _____

☐ Dry   ☐ Humid   ☐ Wet   Allergen Levels: _____

STRESS LEVELS

| None | Low | Medium | High | Max | @$#%! |

FOOD / MEDICATIONS

FOOD / DRINKS	MEDS / SUPPLEMENTS	TIME	DOSE
	☐ usual daily medication		

EXERCISE / DAILY ACTIVITY

☐ Heck yes, I worked out.

☐ I managed to exercise a bit.

☐ No, I haven't exercised at all.

☐ I did some stuff, and that counts.

DETAILS

NOTES / TRIGGERS / IMPROVEMENTS

_____

_____

_____

WRITE ONE THING YOU'RE GRATEFUL FOR

Date:_____

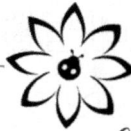

How are you feeling today?

Like death	Terrible	Not good	Meh	Good	Great!	Amazing!

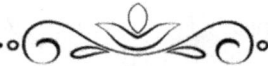

RATE YOUR PAIN LEVEL

① ② ③ ④ ⑤ ⑥ ⑦ ⑧ ⑨ ⑩

Describe your pain / symptoms

	am	pm
_____	☐	☐
_____	☐	☐
_____	☐	☐
_____	☐	☐
_____	☐	☐
_____	☐	☐
_____	☐	☐
_____	☐	☐

Where do you feel it?

Front   Back

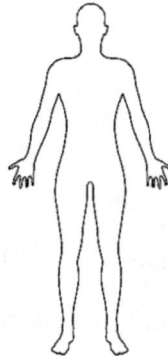

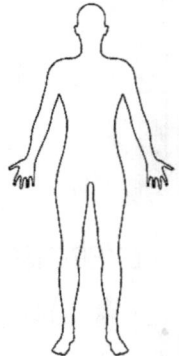

What about your...?

Mood	① ② ③ ④ ⑤ ⑥ ⑦ ⑧ ⑨ ⑩
Energy levels	① ② ③ ④ ⑤ ⑥ ⑦ ⑧ ⑨ ⑩
Mental clarity	① ② ③ ④ ⑤ ⑥ ⑦ ⑧ ⑨ ⑩

Feeling sick?

☐ Nope!

☐ Yes...

☐ Nausea   ☐ Diarrhea   ☐ Vomiting   ☐ Sore throat

☐ Congestion   ☐ Coughing   ☐ Chills   ☐ Fever

Other symptoms: _____

LET'S EXPLORE SOME MORE #25

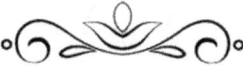

Hours of Sleep ① ② ③ ④ ⑤ ⑥ ⑦ ⑧ ⑨ ⑩ ⊕

Sleep Quality ① ② ③ ④ ⑤ ⑥ ⑦ ⑧ ⑨ ⑩

WEATHER

☐ Hot ☐ Mild ☐ Cold BM Pressure: _____

☐ Dry ☐ Humid ☐ Wet Allergen Levels: _____

STRESS LEVELS

| None | Low | Medium | High | Max | @$#%! |

FOOD / MEDICATIONS

FOOD / DRINKS	MEDS / SUPPLEMENTS	TIME	DOSE
	☐ usual daily medication		

EXERCISE / DAILY ACTIVITY

DETAILS

☐ Heck yes, I worked out.

☐ I managed to exercise a bit.

☐ No, I haven't exercised at all.

☐ I did some stuff, and that counts.

NOTES / TRIGGERS / IMPROVEMENTS

_____

_____

_____

WRITE ONE THING YOU'RE GRATEFUL FOR

_____

Date: _____

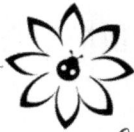

How are you feeling today?

Like death	Terrible	Not good	Meh	Good	Great!	Amazing!

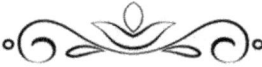

RATE YOUR PAIN LEVEL

(1) (2) (3) (4) (5) (6) (7) (8) (9) (10)

Describe your pain / symptoms

	am	pm
_____	☐	☐
_____	☐	☐
_____	☐	☐
_____	☐	☐
_____	☐	☐
_____	☐	☐
_____	☐	☐
_____	☐	☐

Where do you feel it?

Front   *Back*

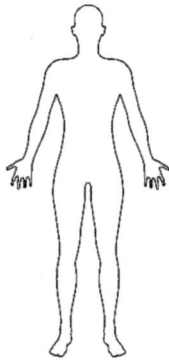

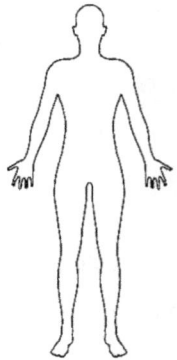

What about your...?

Mood	(1) (2) (3) (4) (5) (6) (7) (8) (9) (10)
Energy levels	(1) (2) (3) (4) (5) (6) (7) (8) (9) (10)
Mental clarity	(1) (2) (3) (4) (5) (6) (7) (8) (9) (10)

Feeling sick?

☐ Nope!

☐ Yes...

☐ Nausea   ☐ Diarrhea   ☐ Vomiting   ☐ Sore throat

☐ Congestion   ☐ Coughing   ☐ Chills   ☐ Fever

Other symptoms: _____

LET'S EXPLORE SOME MORE #26

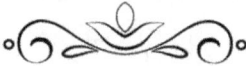

Hours of Sleep ① ② ③ ④ ⑤ ⑥ ⑦ ⑧ ⑨ ⑩ ⊕
Sleep Quality ① ② ③ ④ ⑤ ⑥ ⑦ ⑧ ⑨ ⑩

WEATHER

☐ Hot   ☐ Mild   ☐ Cold   BM Pressure: _____
☐ Dry   ☐ Humid   ☐ Wet   Allergen Levels: _____

STRESS LEVELS

None	Low	Medium	High	Max	@$#%!

FOOD / MEDICATIONS

FOOD / DRINKS	MEDS / SUPPLEMENTS	TIME	DOSE

☐ usual daily medication

EXERCISE / DAILY ACTIVITY

☐ Heck yes, I worked out.
☐ I managed to exercise a bit.
☐ No, I haven't exercised at all.
☐ I did some stuff, and that counts.

DETAILS

NOTES / TRIGGERS / IMPROVEMENTS

WRITE ONE THING YOU'RE GRATEFUL FOR

Date: _____

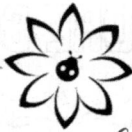

How are you feeling today?

Like death	Terrible	Not good	Meh	Good	Great!	Amazing!

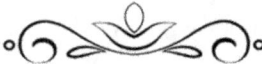

RATE YOUR PAIN LEVEL

① ② ③ ④ ⑤ ⑥ ⑦ ⑧ ⑨ ⑩

Describe your pain / symptoms   Where do you feel it?

	am	pm
	☐	☐
	☐	☐
	☐	☐
	☐	☐
	☐	☐
	☐	☐
	☐	☐
	☐	☐

Front   *Back*

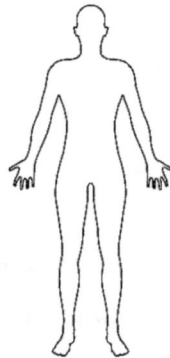 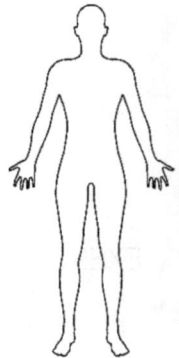

What about your...?   Feeling sick?

Mood   ①②③④⑤⑥⑦⑧⑨⑩   ☐ Nope!

Energy levels ①②③④⑤⑥⑦⑧⑨⑩   ☐ Yes...

Mental clarity ①②③④⑤⑥⑦⑧⑨⑩

☐ Nausea   ☐ Diarrhea   ☐ Vomiting   ☐ Sore throat

☐ Congestion ☐ Coughing   ☐ Chills   ☐ Fever

Other symptoms: _____

LET'S EXPLORE SOME MORE #27

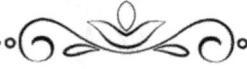

Hours of Sleep ① ② ③ ④ ⑤ ⑥ ⑦ ⑧ ⑨ ⑩ ⊕

Sleep Quality ① ② ③ ④ ⑤ ⑥ ⑦ ⑧ ⑨ ⑩

WEATHER

☐ Hot ☐ Mild ☐ Cold BM Pressure: _____

☐ Dry ☐ Humid ☐ Wet Allergen Levels: _____

STRESS LEVELS

None	Low	Medium	High	Max	@$#%!

FOOD / MEDICATIONS

FOOD / DRINKS	MEDS / SUPPLEMENTS	TIME	DOSE

☐ usual daily medication

EXERCISE / DAILY ACTIVITY

☐ Heck yes, I worked out.

☐ I managed to exercise a bit.

☐ No, I haven't exercised at all.

☐ I did some stuff, and that counts.

DETAILS

NOTES / TRIGGERS / IMPROVEMENTS

_____

_____

_____

WRITE ONE THING YOU'RE GRATEFUL FOR

_____

Date:_____

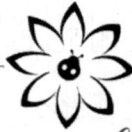

How are you feeling today?

😵 Like death 😣 Terrible 😠 Not good 🙂 Meh 😀 Good 😁 Great! 😍 Amazing!

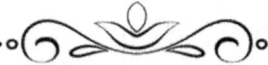

RATE YOUR PAIN LEVEL

① ② ③ ④ ⑤ ⑥ ⑦ ⑧ ⑨ ⑩

Describe your pain / symptoms   Where do you feel it?

	am	pm		
	☐	☐	*Front*	*Back*
	☐	☐		
	☐	☐		
	☐	☐		
	☐	☐		
	☐	☐		
	☐	☐		
	☐	☐		

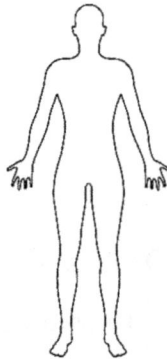 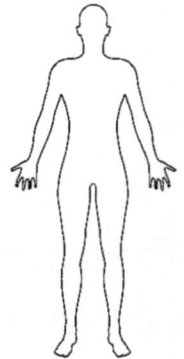

What about your...?   Feeling sick?

Mood   ①②③④⑤⑥⑦⑧⑨⑩   ☐ Nope!
Energy levels   ①②③④⑤⑥⑦⑧⑨⑩   ☐ Yes...
Mental clarity ①②③④⑤⑥⑦⑧⑨⑩

☐ Nausea   ☐ Diarrhea   ☐ Vomiting   ☐ Sore throat
☐ Congestion   ☐ Coughing   ☐ Chills   ☐ Fever

Other symptoms:_____

LET'S EXPLORE SOME MORE #28

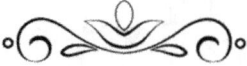

Hours of Sleep (1) (2) (3) (4) (5) (6) (7) (8) (9) (10) (+)

Sleep Quality (1) (2) (3) (4) (5) (6) (7) (8) (9) (10)

WEATHER

☐ Hot ☐ Mild ☐ Cold BM Pressure: _____

☐ Dry ☐ Humid ☐ Wet Allergen Levels: _____

STRESS LEVELS

None	Low	Medium	High	Max	@$#%!

FOOD / MEDICATIONS

FOOD / DRINKS	MEDS / SUPPLEMENTS	TIME	DOSE

☐ usual daily medication

EXERCISE / DAILY ACTIVITY

☐ Heck yes, I worked out.

☐ I managed to exercise a bit.

☐ No, I haven't exercised at all.

☐ I did some stuff, and that counts.

DETAILS

NOTES / TRIGGERS / IMPROVEMENTS

_____

_____

_____

WRITE ONE THING YOU'RE GRATEFUL FOR

_____

Date: _____

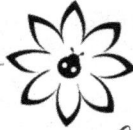

How are you feeling today?

| Like death | Terrible | Not good | Meh | Good | Great! | Amazing! |

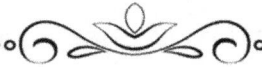

RATE YOUR PAIN LEVEL

① ② ③ ④ ⑤ ⑥ ⑦ ⑧ ⑨ ⑩

Describe your pain / symptoms

Where do you feel it?

	am	pm
	☐	☐
	☐	☐
	☐	☐
	☐	☐
	☐	☐
	☐	☐
	☐	☐
	☐	☐

Front   *Back*

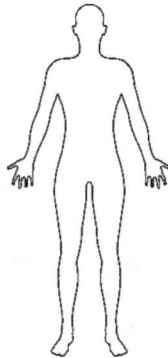

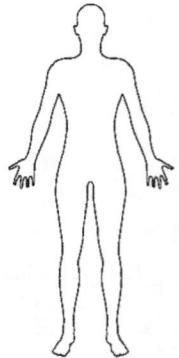

What about your...?

Feeling sick?

Mood   ① ② ③ ④ ⑤ ⑥ ⑦ ⑧ ⑨ ⑩   ☐ Nope!
Energy levels   ① ② ③ ④ ⑤ ⑥ ⑦ ⑧ ⑨ ⑩   ☐ Yes...
Mental clarity ① ② ③ ④ ⑤ ⑥ ⑦ ⑧ ⑨ ⑩

☐ Nausea   ☐ Diarrhea   ☐ Vomiting   ☐ Sore throat
☐ Congestion   ☐ Coughing   ☐ Chills   ☐ Fever

Other symptoms: _____

LET'S EXPLORE SOME MORE

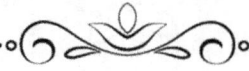

| Hours of Sleep | ① ② ③ ④ ⑤ ⑥ ⑦ ⑧ ⑨ ⑩ ⊕ |
| Sleep Quality | ① ② ③ ④ ⑤ ⑥ ⑦ ⑧ ⑨ ⑩ |

WEATHER

☐ Hot   ☐ Mild   ☐ Cold   BM Pressure: _____

☐ Dry   ☐ Humid   ☐ Wet   Allergen Levels: _____

STRESS LEVELS

| None | Low | Medium | High | Max | @$#%! |

FOOD / MEDICATIONS

FOOD / DRINKS	MEDS / SUPPLEMENTS	TIME	DOSE

☐ usual daily medication

EXERCISE / DAILY ACTIVITY

☐ Heck yes, I worked out.

☐ I managed to exercise a bit.

☐ No, I haven't exercised at all.

☐ I did some stuff, and that counts.

DETAILS

NOTES / TRIGGERS / IMPROVEMENTS

WRITE ONE THING YOU'RE GRATEFUL FOR

Date: _____

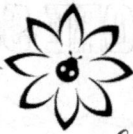

How are you feeling today?

| Like death | Terrible | Not good | Meh | Good | Great! | Amazing! |

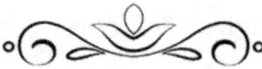

RATE YOUR PAIN LEVEL

① ② ③ ④ ⑤ ⑥ ⑦ ⑧ ⑨ ⑩

Describe your pain / symptoms

Where do you feel it?

	am	pm
	☐	☐
	☐	☐
	☐	☐
	☐	☐
	☐	☐
	☐	☐
	☐	☐
	☐	☐

Front *Back*

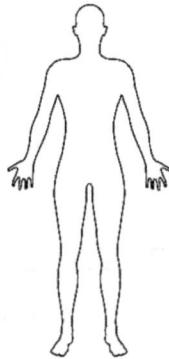 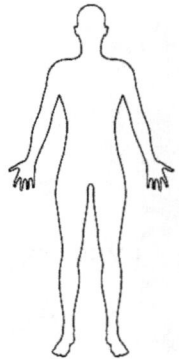

What about your...?

Feeling sick?

Mood ① ② ③ ④ ⑤ ⑥ ⑦ ⑧ ⑨ ⑩   ☐ Nope!

Energy levels ① ② ③ ④ ⑤ ⑥ ⑦ ⑧ ⑨ ⑩   ☐ Yes...

Mental clarity ① ② ③ ④ ⑤ ⑥ ⑦ ⑧ ⑨ ⑩

☐ Nausea   ☐ Diarrhea   ☐ Vomiting   ☐ Sore throat

☐ Congestion   ☐ Coughing   ☐ Chills   ☐ Fever

Other symptoms: _____

LET'S EXPLORE SOME MORE #30

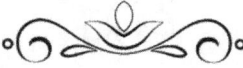

Hours of Sleep ① ② ③ ④ ⑤ ⑥ ⑦ ⑧ ⑨ ⑩ ⊕

Sleep Quality ① ② ③ ④ ⑤ ⑥ ⑦ ⑧ ⑨ ⑩

WEATHER

☐ Hot ☐ Mild ☐ Cold BM Pressure: _____

☐ Dry ☐ Humid ☐ Wet Allergen Levels: _____

STRESS LEVELS

None	Low	Medium	High	Max	@$#%!

FOOD / MEDICATIONS

FOOD / DRINKS	MEDS / SUPPLEMENTS	TIME	DOSE

☐ usual daily medication

EXERCISE / DAILY ACTIVITY

☐ Heck yes, I worked out.

☐ I managed to exercise a bit.

☐ No, I haven't exercised at all.

☐ I did some stuff, and that counts.

DETAILS

NOTES / TRIGGERS / IMPROVEMENTS

_____

_____

_____

WRITE ONE THING YOU'RE GRATEFUL FOR

_____

Date: _____

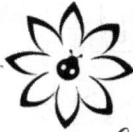

How are you feeling today?

Like death	Terrible	Not good	Meh	Good	Great!	Amazing!

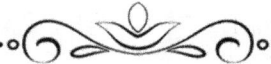

RATE YOUR PAIN LEVEL

(1) (2) (3) (4) (5) (6) (7) (8) (9) (10)

Describe your pain / symptoms

	am	pm
	☐	☐
	☐	☐
	☐	☐
	☐	☐
	☐	☐
	☐	☐
	☐	☐
	☐	☐

Where do you feel it?

Front   *Back*

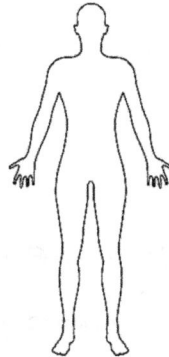

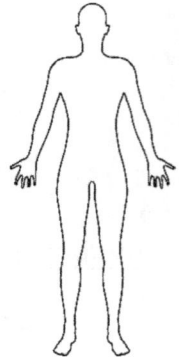

What about your...?

Mood   (1) (2) (3) (4) (5) (6) (7) (8) (9) (10)
Energy levels   (1) (2) (3) (4) (5) (6) (7) (8) (9) (10)
Mental clarity (1) (2) (3) (4) (5) (6) (7) (8) (9) (10)

Feeling sick?

☐ Nope!
☐ Yes...

☐ Nausea   ☐ Diarrhea   ☐ Vomiting   ☐ Sore throat
☐ Congestion ☐ Coughing   ☐ Chills   ☐ Fever

Other symptoms: _____

LET'S EXPLORE SOME MORE #31

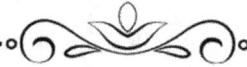

Hours of Sleep	① ② ③ ④ ⑤ ⑥ ⑦ ⑧ ⑨ ⑩ ⊕
Sleep Quality	① ② ③ ④ ⑤ ⑥ ⑦ ⑧ ⑨ ⑩

WEATHER

☐ Hot ☐ Mild ☐ Cold BM Pressure: _____

☐ Dry ☐ Humid ☐ Wet Allergen Levels: _____

STRESS LEVELS

None	Low	Medium	High	Max	@$#%!

FOOD / MEDICATIONS

FOOD / DRINKS	MEDS / SUPPLEMENTS	TIME	DOSE
	☐ usual daily medication		

EXERCISE / DAILY ACTIVITY

☐ Heck yes, I worked out.

☐ I managed to exercise a bit.

☐ No, I haven't exercised at all.

☐ I did some stuff, and that counts.

DETAILS

NOTES / TRIGGERS / IMPROVEMENTS

_____

_____

_____

WRITE ONE THING YOU'RE GRATEFUL FOR

_____

Date:_____

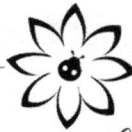

How are you feeling today?

| Like death | Terrible | Not good | Meh | Good | Great! | Amazing! |

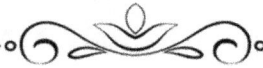

RATE YOUR PAIN LEVEL

(1) (2) (3) (4) (5) (6) (7) (8) (9) (10)

Describe your pain / symptoms   Where do you feel it?

	am	pm	Front	Back
_____	☐	☐		
_____	☐	☐		
_____	☐	☐		
_____	☐	☐		
_____	☐	☐		
_____	☐	☐		
_____	☐	☐		
_____	☐	☐		

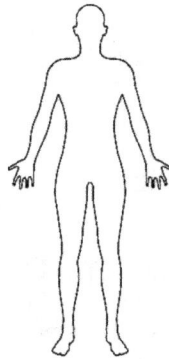

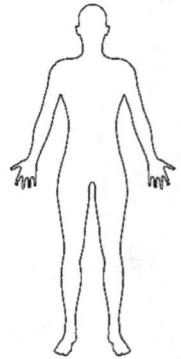

What about your...?   Feeling sick?

Mood   (1)(2)(3)(4)(5)(6)(7)(8)(9)(10)   ☐ Nope!

Energy levels   (1)(2)(3)(4)(5)(6)(7)(8)(9)(10)   ☐ Yes...

Mental clarity (1)(2)(3)(4)(5)(6)(7)(8)(9)(10)

☐ Nausea   ☐ Diarrhea   ☐ Vomiting   ☐ Sore throat

☐ Congestion   ☐ Coughing   ☐ Chills   ☐ Fever

Other symptoms: _____

LET'S EXPLORE SOME MORE   #32

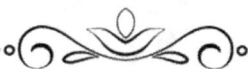

Hours of Sleep   ① ② ③ ④ ⑤ ⑥ ⑦ ⑧ ⑨ ⑩ ⊕
Sleep Quality   ① ② ③ ④ ⑤ ⑥ ⑦ ⑧ ⑨ ⑩

WEATHER

☐ Hot   ☐ Mild   ☐ Cold   BM Pressure: _____

☐ Dry   ☐ Humid   ☐ Wet   Allergen Levels: _____

STRESS LEVELS

None	Low	Medium	High	Max	@$#%!

FOOD / MEDICATIONS

FOOD / DRINKS	MEDS / SUPPLEMENTS	TIME	DOSE

☐ usual daily medication

EXERCISE / DAILY ACTIVITY

☐ Heck yes, I worked out.

☐ I managed to exercise a bit.

☐ No, I haven't exercised at all.

☐ I did some stuff, and that counts.

DETAILS

NOTES / TRIGGERS / IMPROVEMENTS

WRITE ONE THING YOU'RE GRATEFUL FOR

Date: _____

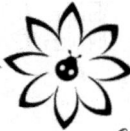

How are you feeling today?

😵 Like death   😣 Terrible   😠 Not good   🙂 Meh   😊 Good   😁 Great!   😍 Amazing!

RATE YOUR PAIN LEVEL

① ② ③ ④ ⑤ ⑥ ⑦ ⑧ ⑨ ⑩

Describe your pain / symptoms

	am	pm
	☐	☐
	☐	☐
	☐	☐
	☐	☐
	☐	☐
	☐	☐
	☐	☐
	☐	☐

Where do you feel it?

Front   *Back*

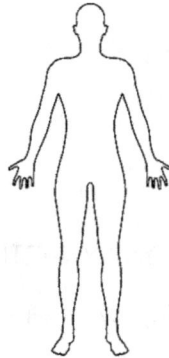 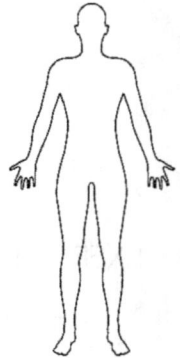

What about your...?

Mood ① ② ③ ④ ⑤ ⑥ ⑦ ⑧ ⑨ ⑩

Energy levels ① ② ③ ④ ⑤ ⑥ ⑦ ⑧ ⑨ ⑩

Mental clarity ① ② ③ ④ ⑤ ⑥ ⑦ ⑧ ⑨ ⑩

Feeling sick?

☐ Nope!

☐ Yes...

☐ Nausea   ☐ Diarrhea   ☐ Vomiting   ☐ Sore throat

☐ Congestion   ☐ Coughing   ☐ Chills   ☐ Fever

Other symptoms: _____

LET'S EXPLORE SOME MORE #33

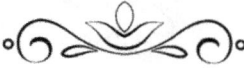

Hours of Sleep ① ② ③ ④ ⑤ ⑥ ⑦ ⑧ ⑨ ⑩ ⊕

Sleep Quality ① ② ③ ④ ⑤ ⑥ ⑦ ⑧ ⑨ ⑩

WEATHER

☐ Hot ☐ Mild ☐ Cold BM Pressure: _____

☐ Dry ☐ Humid ☐ Wet Allergen Levels: _____

STRESS LEVELS

None	Low	Medium	High	Max	@$#%!

FOOD / MEDICATIONS

FOOD / DRINKS	MEDS / SUPPLEMENTS	TIME	DOSE

☐ usual daily medication

EXERCISE / DAILY ACTIVITY

☐ Heck yes, I worked out.

☐ I managed to exercise a bit.

☐ No, I haven't exercised at all.

☐ I did some stuff, and that counts.

DETAILS

NOTES / TRIGGERS / IMPROVEMENTS

_____

_____

_____

WRITE ONE THING YOU'RE GRATEFUL FOR

Date: _____

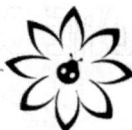

How are you feeling today?

| Like death | Terrible | Not good | Meh | Good | Great! | Amazing! |

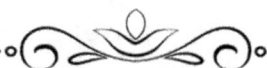

RATE YOUR PAIN LEVEL

(1) (2) (3) (4) (5) (6) (7) (8) (9) (10)

Describe your pain / symptoms

	am	pm
_____	☐	☐
_____	☐	☐
_____	☐	☐
_____	☐	☐
_____	☐	☐
_____	☐	☐
_____	☐	☐
_____	☐	☐

Where do you feel it?

Front   *Back*

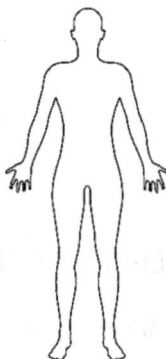

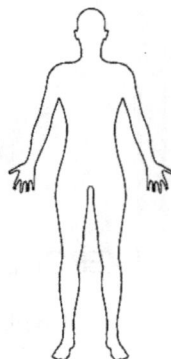

What about your...?

Mood	(1) (2) (3) (4) (5) (6) (7) (8) (9) (10)
Energy levels	(1) (2) (3) (4) (5) (6) (7) (8) (9) (10)
Mental clarity	(1) (2) (3) (4) (5) (6) (7) (8) (9) (10)

Feeling sick?

☐ Nope!

☐ Yes...

☐ Nausea   ☐ Diarrhea   ☐ Vomiting   ☐ Sore throat

☐ Congestion   ☐ Coughing   ☐ Chills   ☐ Fever

Other symptoms: _____

LET'S EXPLORE SOME MORE #34

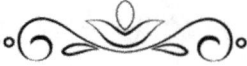

Hours of Sleep ① ② ③ ④ ⑤ ⑥ ⑦ ⑧ ⑨ ⑩ ⊕

Sleep Quality ① ② ③ ④ ⑤ ⑥ ⑦ ⑧ ⑨ ⑩

WEATHER

☐ Hot   ☐ Mild   ☐ Cold   BM Pressure: _____

☐ Dry   ☐ Humid   ☐ Wet   Allergen Levels: _____

STRESS LEVELS

None	Low	Medium	High	Max	@$#%!

FOOD / MEDICATIONS

FOOD / DRINKS	MEDS / SUPPLEMENTS	TIME	DOSE

☐ usual daily medication

EXERCISE / DAILY ACTIVITY

☐ Heck yes, I worked out.

☐ I managed to exercise a bit.

☐ No, I haven't exercised at all.

☐ I did some stuff, and that counts.

DETAILS

NOTES / TRIGGERS / IMPROVEMENTS

WRITE ONE THING YOU'RE GRATEFUL FOR

Date: _____

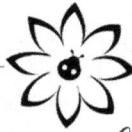

How are you feeling today?

Like death	Terrible	Not good	Meh	Good	Great!	Amazing!

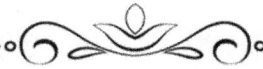

RATE YOUR PAIN LEVEL

(1) (2) (3) (4) (5) (6) (7) (8) (9) (10)

Describe your pain / symptoms

	am	pm
_____	☐	☐
_____	☐	☐
_____	☐	☐
_____	☐	☐
_____	☐	☐
_____	☐	☐
_____	☐	☐
_____	☐	☐

Where do you feel it?

Front   *Back*

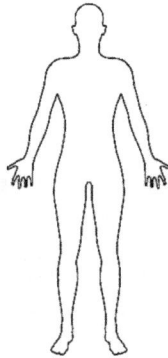

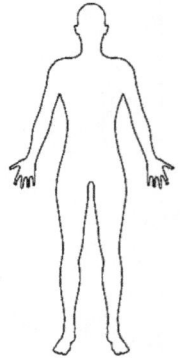

What about your...?

Mood	(1) (2) (3) (4) (5) (6) (7) (8) (9) (10)
Energy levels	(1) (2) (3) (4) (5) (6) (7) (8) (9) (10)
Mental clarity	(1) (2) (3) (4) (5) (6) (7) (8) (9) (10)

Feeling sick?

☐ Nope!
☐ Yes...

☐ Nausea   ☐ Diarrhea   ☐ Vomiting   ☐ Sore throat
☐ Congestion   ☐ Coughing   ☐ Chills   ☐ Fever

Other symptoms: _____

LET'S EXPLORE SOME MORE #35

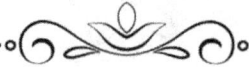

Hours of Sleep (1) (2) (3) (4) (5) (6) (7) (8) (9) (10) (+)

Sleep Quality (1) (2) (3) (4) (5) (6) (7) (8) (9) (10)

WEATHER

☐ Hot   ☐ Mild   ☐ Cold   BM Pressure: _____

☐ Dry   ☐ Humid   ☐ Wet   Allergen Levels: _____

STRESS LEVELS

None	Low	Medium	High	Max	@$#%!

FOOD / MEDICATIONS

FOOD / DRINKS	MEDS / SUPPLEMENTS	TIME	DOSE

☐ usual daily medication

EXERCISE / DAILY ACTIVITY

☐ Heck yes, I worked out.

☐ I managed to exercise a bit.

☐ No, I haven't exercised at all.

☐ I did some stuff, and that counts.

DETAILS

NOTES / TRIGGERS / IMPROVEMENTS

_____

_____

_____

WRITE ONE THING YOU'RE GRATEFUL FOR

_____

Date: _____

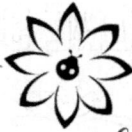

How are you feeling today?

😵	😖	😠	😐	🙂	😁	😍
Like death	Terrible	Not good	Meh	Good	Great!	Amazing!

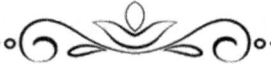

RATE YOUR PAIN LEVEL

① ② ③ ④ ⑤ ⑥ ⑦ ⑧ ⑨ ⑩

Describe your pain / symptoms   Where do you feel it?

	am	pm
	☐	☐
	☐	☐
	☐	☐
	☐	☐
	☐	☐
	☐	☐
	☐	☐
	☐	☐

Front   *Back*

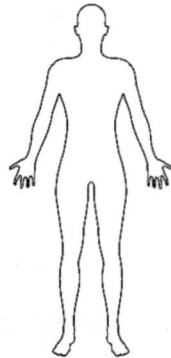
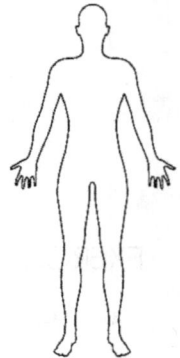

What about your…?   Feeling sick?

Mood	① ② ③ ④ ⑤ ⑥ ⑦ ⑧ ⑨ ⑩
Energy levels	① ② ③ ④ ⑤ ⑥ ⑦ ⑧ ⑨ ⑩
Mental clarity	① ② ③ ④ ⑤ ⑥ ⑦ ⑧ ⑨ ⑩

☐ Nope!
☐ Yes…

☐ Nausea   ☐ Diarrhea   ☐ Vomiting   ☐ Sore throat
☐ Congestion   ☐ Coughing   ☐ Chills   ☐ Fever

Other symptoms: _____

LET'S EXPLORE SOME MORE   #36

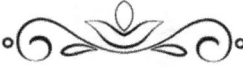

| Hours of Sleep | ① ② ③ ④ ⑤ ⑥ ⑦ ⑧ ⑨ ⑩ ⊕ |
| Sleep Quality | ① ② ③ ④ ⑤ ⑥ ⑦ ⑧ ⑨ ⑩ |

WEATHER

☐ Hot ☐ Mild ☐ Cold   BM Pressure: _____

☐ Dry ☐ Humid ☐ Wet   Allergen Levels: _____

STRESS LEVELS

| None | Low | Medium | High | Max | @$#%! |

FOOD / MEDICATIONS

FOOD / DRINKS	MEDS / SUPPLEMENTS	TIME	DOSE

☐ usual daily medication

EXERCISE / DAILY ACTIVITY

☐ Heck yes, I worked out.

☐ I managed to exercise a bit.

☐ No, I haven't exercised at all.

☐ I did some stuff, and that counts.

DETAILS

NOTES / TRIGGERS / IMPROVEMENTS

WRITE ONE THING YOU'RE GRATEFUL FOR

Date: _____

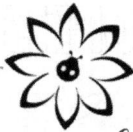

How are you feeling today?

| Like death | Terrible | Not good | Meh | Good | Great! | Amazing! |

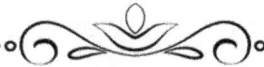

RATE YOUR PAIN LEVEL

(1) (2) (3) (4) (5) (6) (7) (8) (9) (10)

Describe your pain / symptoms   Where do you feel it?

	am	pm
	☐	☐
	☐	☐
	☐	☐
	☐	☐
	☐	☐
	☐	☐
	☐	☐
	☐	☐

Front   *Back*

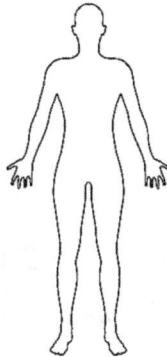

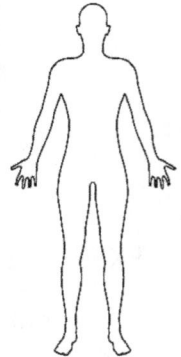

What about your...?   Feeling sick?

Mood   (1)(2)(3)(4)(5)(6)(7)(8)(9)(10)   ☐ Nope!
Energy levels   (1)(2)(3)(4)(5)(6)(7)(8)(9)(10)   ☐ Yes...
Mental clarity (1)(2)(3)(4)(5)(6)(7)(8)(9)(10)

☐ Nausea   ☐ Diarrhea   ☐ Vomiting   ☐ Sore throat
☐ Congestion   ☐ Coughing   ☐ Chills   ☐ Fever

Other symptoms: _____

LET'S EXPLORE SOME MORE #37

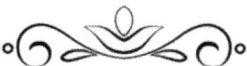

Hours of Sleep ① ② ③ ④ ⑤ ⑥ ⑦ ⑧ ⑨ ⑩ ⊕

Sleep Quality ① ② ③ ④ ⑤ ⑥ ⑦ ⑧ ⑨ ⑩

WEATHER

☐ Hot ☐ Mild ☐ Cold BM Pressure: _____

☐ Dry ☐ Humid ☐ Wet Allergen Levels: _____

STRESS LEVELS

None	Low	Medium	High	Max	@$#%!

FOOD / MEDICATIONS

FOOD / DRINKS	MEDS / SUPPLEMENTS	TIME	DOSE

☐ usual daily medication

EXERCISE / DAILY ACTIVITY

☐ Heck yes, I worked out.

☐ I managed to exercise a bit.

☐ No, I haven't exercised at all.

☐ I did some stuff, and that counts.

DETAILS

NOTES / TRIGGERS / IMPROVEMENTS

WRITE ONE THING YOU'RE GRATEFUL FOR

Date:_____

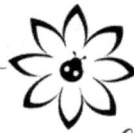

How are you feeling today?

| Like death | Terrible | Not good | Meh | Good | Great! | Amazing! |

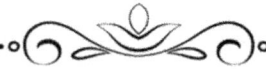

RATE YOUR PAIN LEVEL

(1) (2) (3) (4) (5) (6) (7) (8) (9) (10)

Describe your pain / symptoms

	am	pm
_____	☐	☐
_____	☐	☐
_____	☐	☐
_____	☐	☐
_____	☐	☐
_____	☐	☐
_____	☐	☐
_____	☐	☐

Where do you feel it?

Front   *Back*

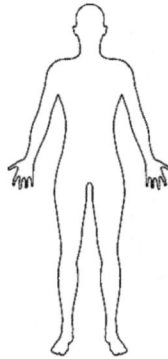

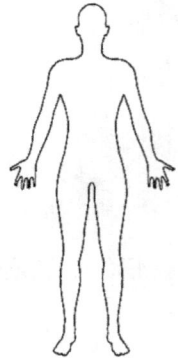

What about your...?

Mood	(1) (2) (3) (4) (5) (6) (7) (8) (9) (10)
Energy levels	(1) (2) (3) (4) (5) (6) (7) (8) (9) (10)
Mental clarity	(1) (2) (3) (4) (5) (6) (7) (8) (9) (10)

Feeling sick?

☐ Nope!

☐ Yes...

☐ Nausea   ☐ Diarrhea   ☐ Vomiting   ☐ Sore throat

☐ Congestion   ☐ Coughing   ☐ Chills   ☐ Fever

Other symptoms: _____

LET'S EXPLORE SOME MORE #38

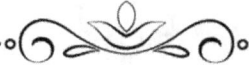

Hours of Sleep ① ② ③ ④ ⑤ ⑥ ⑦ ⑧ ⑨ ⑩ ⊕

Sleep Quality ① ② ③ ④ ⑤ ⑥ ⑦ ⑧ ⑨ ⑩

WEATHER

☐ Hot   ☐ Mild   ☐ Cold   BM Pressure: _____

☐ Dry   ☐ Humid   ☐ Wet   Allergen Levels: _____

STRESS LEVELS

None	Low	Medium	High	Max	@$#%!

FOOD / MEDICATIONS

FOOD / DRINKS	MEDS / SUPPLEMENTS	TIME	DOSE

☐ usual daily medication

EXERCISE / DAILY ACTIVITY

☐ Heck yes, I worked out.

☐ I managed to exercise a bit.

☐ No, I haven't exercised at all.

☐ I did some stuff, and that counts.

DETAILS

NOTES / TRIGGERS / IMPROVEMENTS

WRITE ONE THING YOU'RE GRATEFUL FOR

Date:_____

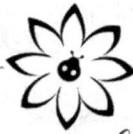

How are you feeling today?

Like death	Terrible	Not good	Meh	Good	Great!	Amazing!

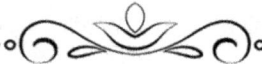

RATE YOUR PAIN LEVEL

① ② ③ ④ ⑤ ⑥ ⑦ ⑧ ⑨ ⑩

Describe your pain / symptoms

Where do you feel it?

	am	pm
	☐	☐
	☐	☐
	☐	☐
	☐	☐
	☐	☐
	☐	☐
	☐	☐
	☐	☐

Front   *Back*

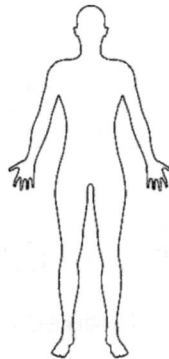 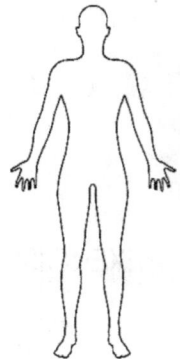

What about your...?

Feeling sick?

Mood	① ② ③ ④ ⑤ ⑥ ⑦ ⑧ ⑨ ⑩	☐ Nope!
Energy levels	① ② ③ ④ ⑤ ⑥ ⑦ ⑧ ⑨ ⑩	☐ Yes...
Mental clarity	① ② ③ ④ ⑤ ⑥ ⑦ ⑧ ⑨ ⑩	

☐ Nausea   ☐ Diarrhea   ☐ Vomiting   ☐ Sore throat

☐ Congestion   ☐ Coughing   ☐ Chills   ☐ Fever

Other symptoms: _____

LET'S EXPLORE SOME MORE #39

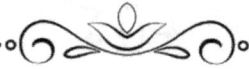

Hours of Sleep ① ② ③ ④ ⑤ ⑥ ⑦ ⑧ ⑨ ⑩ ⊕
Sleep Quality ① ② ③ ④ ⑤ ⑥ ⑦ ⑧ ⑨ ⑩

WEATHER

☐ Hot ☐ Mild ☐ Cold BM Pressure: _____
☐ Dry ☐ Humid ☐ Wet Allergen Levels: _____

STRESS LEVELS

None	Low	Medium	High	Max	@$#%!

FOOD / MEDICATIONS

FOOD / DRINKS	MEDS / SUPPLEMENTS	TIME	DOSE

☐ usual daily medication

EXERCISE / DAILY ACTIVITY

☐ Heck yes, I worked out.
☐ I managed to exercise a bit.
☐ No, I haven't exercised at all.
☐ I did some stuff, and that counts.

DETAILS

NOTES / TRIGGERS / IMPROVEMENTS

WRITE ONE THING YOU'RE GRATEFUL FOR

Date: _____

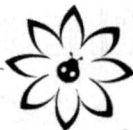

How are you feeling today?

😵 Like death 😣 Terrible 😠 Not good 🙂 Meh 😊 Good 😁 Great! 🥰 Amazing!

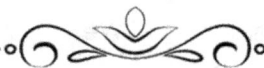

RATE YOUR PAIN LEVEL

① ② ③ ④ ⑤ ⑥ ⑦ ⑧ ⑨ ⑩

Describe your pain / symptoms

	am	pm
	☐	☐
	☐	☐
	☐	☐
	☐	☐
	☐	☐
	☐	☐
	☐	☐
	☐	☐

Where do you feel it?

Front   *Back*

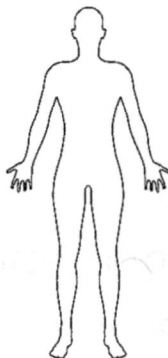 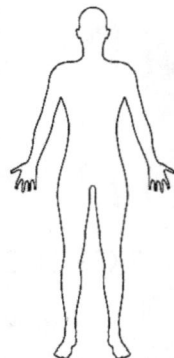

What about your...?

Mood ① ② ③ ④ ⑤ ⑥ ⑦ ⑧ ⑨ ⑩

Energy levels ① ② ③ ④ ⑤ ⑥ ⑦ ⑧ ⑨ ⑩

Mental clarity ① ② ③ ④ ⑤ ⑥ ⑦ ⑧ ⑨ ⑩

Feeling sick?

☐ Nope!

☐ Yes...

☐ Nausea   ☐ Diarrhea   ☐ Vomiting   ☐ Sore throat

☐ Congestion   ☐ Coughing   ☐ Chills   ☐ Fever

Other symptoms: _____

LET'S EXPLORE SOME MORE #40

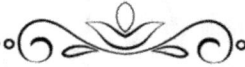

Hours of Sleep ① ② ③ ④ ⑤ ⑥ ⑦ ⑧ ⑨ ⑩ (+)

Sleep Quality ① ② ③ ④ ⑤ ⑥ ⑦ ⑧ ⑨ ⑩

WEATHER

☐ Hot ☐ Mild ☐ Cold BM Pressure: _____

☐ Dry ☐ Humid ☐ Wet Allergen Levels: _____

STRESS LEVELS

None	Low	Medium	High	Max	@$#%!

FOOD / MEDICATIONS

FOOD / DRINKS	MEDS / SUPPLEMENTS	TIME	DOSE

☐ usual daily medication

EXERCISE / DAILY ACTIVITY

☐ Heck yes, I worked out.

☐ I managed to exercise a bit.

☐ No, I haven't exercised at all.

☐ I did some stuff, and that counts.

DETAILS

NOTES / TRIGGERS / IMPROVEMENTS

_____

_____

_____

WRITE ONE THING YOU'RE GRATEFUL FOR

_____

Date:_____

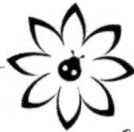

How are you feeling today?

Like death	Terrible	Not good	Meh	Good	Great!	Amazing!

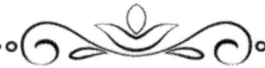

RATE YOUR PAIN LEVEL

① ② ③ ④ ⑤ ⑥ ⑦ ⑧ ⑨ ⑩

Describe your pain / symptoms

	am	pm
	☐	☐
	☐	☐
	☐	☐
	☐	☐
	☐	☐
	☐	☐
	☐	☐
	☐	☐

Where do you feel it?

Front   Back

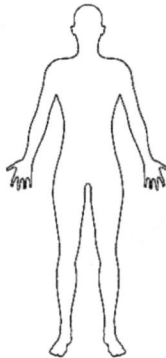

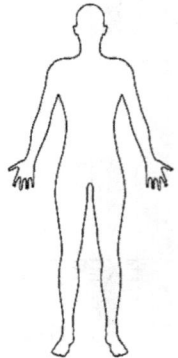

What about your...?

Mood	① ② ③ ④ ⑤ ⑥ ⑦ ⑧ ⑨ ⑩
Energy levels	① ② ③ ④ ⑤ ⑥ ⑦ ⑧ ⑨ ⑩
Mental clarity	① ② ③ ④ ⑤ ⑥ ⑦ ⑧ ⑨ ⑩

Feeling sick?

☐ Nope!
☐ Yes...

☐ Nausea   ☐ Diarrhea   ☐ Vomiting   ☐ Sore throat
☐ Congestion ☐ Coughing   ☐ Chills   ☐ Fever

Other symptoms: _____

LET'S EXPLORE SOME MORE #41

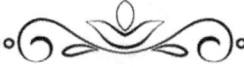

Hours of Sleep ① ② ③ ④ ⑤ ⑥ ⑦ ⑧ ⑨ ⑩ ⊕

Sleep Quality ① ② ③ ④ ⑤ ⑥ ⑦ ⑧ ⑨ ⑩

WEATHER

☐ Hot   ☐ Mild   ☐ Cold   BM Pressure: _____

☐ Dry   ☐ Humid   ☐ Wet   Allergen Levels: _____

STRESS LEVELS

None	Low	Medium	High	Max	@$#%!

FOOD / MEDICATIONS

FOOD / DRINKS	MEDS / SUPPLEMENTS	TIME	DOSE

☐ usual daily medication

EXERCISE / DAILY ACTIVITY

☐ Heck yes, I worked out.

☐ I managed to exercise a bit.

☐ No, I haven't exercised at all.

☐ I did some stuff, and that counts.

DETAILS

NOTES / TRIGGERS / IMPROVEMENTS

WRITE ONE THING YOU'RE GRATEFUL FOR

Date:_____

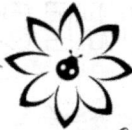

How are you feeling today?

| Like death | Terrible | Not good | Meh | Good | Great! | Amazing! |

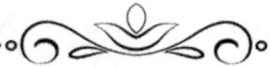

RATE YOUR PAIN LEVEL

① ② ③ ④ ⑤ ⑥ ⑦ ⑧ ⑨ ⑩

Describe your pain / symptoms   Where do you feel it?

	am	pm	Front	Back
	☐	☐		
	☐	☐		
	☐	☐		
	☐	☐		
	☐	☐		
	☐	☐		
	☐	☐		
	☐	☐		

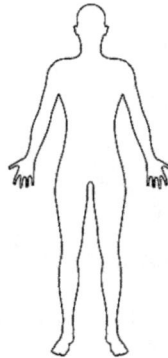

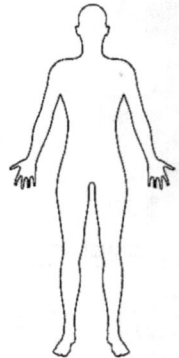

What about your...?   Feeling sick?

Mood   ① ② ③ ④ ⑤ ⑥ ⑦ ⑧ ⑨ ⑩   ☐ Nope!

Energy levels   ① ② ③ ④ ⑤ ⑥ ⑦ ⑧ ⑨ ⑩   ☐ Yes...

Mental clarity ① ② ③ ④ ⑤ ⑥ ⑦ ⑧ ⑨ ⑩

☐ Nausea   ☐ Diarrhea   ☐ Vomiting   ☐ Sore throat

☐ Congestion   ☐ Coughing   ☐ Chills   ☐ Fever

Other symptoms: _____

LET'S EXPLORE SOME MORE #42

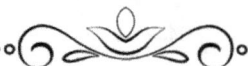

Hours of Sleep ① ② ③ ④ ⑤ ⑥ ⑦ ⑧ ⑨ ⑩ ⊕

Sleep Quality ① ② ③ ④ ⑤ ⑥ ⑦ ⑧ ⑨ ⑩

WEATHER

☐ Hot ☐ Mild ☐ Cold BM Pressure: _____

☐ Dry ☐ Humid ☐ Wet Allergen Levels: _____

STRESS LEVELS

| None | Low | Medium | High | Max | @$#%! |

FOOD / MEDICATIONS

FOOD / DRINKS	MEDS / SUPPLEMENTS	TIME	DOSE

☐ usual daily medication

EXERCISE / DAILY ACTIVITY

☐ Heck yes, I worked out.

☐ I managed to exercise a bit.

☐ No, I haven't exercised at all.

☐ I did some stuff, and that counts.

DETAILS

NOTES / TRIGGERS / IMPROVEMENTS

WRITE ONE THING YOU'RE GRATEFUL FOR

Date:_____

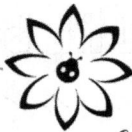

How are you feeling today?

| Like death | Terrible | Not good | Meh | Good | Great! | Amazing! |

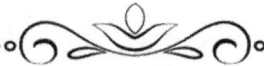

RATE YOUR PAIN LEVEL

① ② ③ ④ ⑤ ⑥ ⑦ ⑧ ⑨ ⑩

Describe your pain / symptoms

Where do you feel it?

	am	pm
	☐	☐
	☐	☐
	☐	☐
	☐	☐
	☐	☐
	☐	☐
	☐	☐
	☐	☐

Front   *Back*

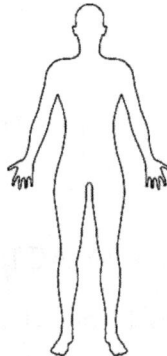

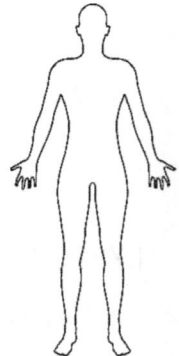

What about your...?

Feeling sick?

Mood	① ② ③ ④ ⑤ ⑥ ⑦ ⑧ ⑨ ⑩	☐ Nope!
Energy levels	① ② ③ ④ ⑤ ⑥ ⑦ ⑧ ⑨ ⑩	☐ Yes...
Mental clarity	① ② ③ ④ ⑤ ⑥ ⑦ ⑧ ⑨ ⑩	

☐ Nausea   ☐ Diarrhea   ☐ Vomiting   ☐ Sore throat

☐ Congestion   ☐ Coughing   ☐ Chills   ☐ Fever

Other symptoms: _____

LET'S EXPLORE SOME MORE #43

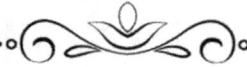

Hours of Sleep (1)(2)(3)(4)(5)(6)(7)(8)(9)(10)(+)

Sleep Quality (1)(2)(3)(4)(5)(6)(7)(8)(9)(10)

WEATHER

☐ Hot   ☐ Mild   ☐ Cold   BM Pressure: _____

☐ Dry   ☐ Humid   ☐ Wet   Allergen Levels: _____

STRESS LEVELS

| None | Low | Medium | High | Max | @$#%! |

FOOD / MEDICATIONS

FOOD / DRINKS	MEDS / SUPPLEMENTS	TIME	DOSE

☐ usual daily medication

EXERCISE / DAILY ACTIVITY

☐ Heck yes, I worked out.

☐ I managed to exercise a bit.

☐ No, I haven't exercised at all.

☐ I did some stuff, and that counts.

DETAILS

NOTES / TRIGGERS / IMPROVEMENTS

_____

_____

_____

WRITE ONE THING YOU'RE GRATEFUL FOR

_____

Date: _____

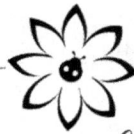

How are you feeling today?

Like death	Terrible	Not good	Meh	Good	Great!	Amazing!

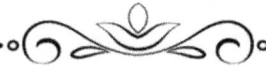

RATE YOUR PAIN LEVEL

(1) (2) (3) (4) (5) (6) (7) (8) (9) (10)

Describe your pain / symptoms

Where do you feel it?

am	pm
☐	☐
☐	☐
☐	☐
☐	☐
☐	☐
☐	☐
☐	☐
☐	☐

Front   *Back*

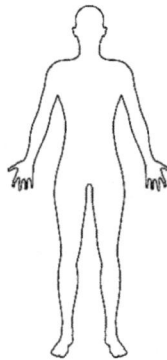

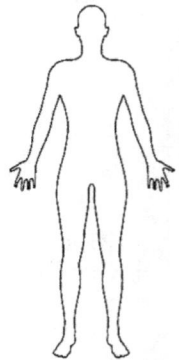

What about your...?

Feeling sick?

Mood	(1)(2)(3)(4)(5)(6)(7)(8)(9)(10)	☐ Nope!
Energy levels	(1)(2)(3)(4)(5)(6)(7)(8)(9)(10)	☐ Yes...
Mental clarity	(1)(2)(3)(4)(5)(6)(7)(8)(9)(10)	

☐ Nausea   ☐ Diarrhea   ☐ Vomiting   ☐ Sore throat

☐ Congestion   ☐ Coughing   ☐ Chills   ☐ Fever

Other symptoms: _____

LET'S EXPLORE SOME MORE #44

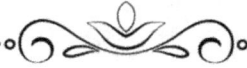

Hours of Sleep (1) (2) (3) (4) (5) (6) (7) (8) (9) (10) (+)

Sleep Quality (1) (2) (3) (4) (5) (6) (7) (8) (9) (10)

WEATHER

☐ Hot ☐ Mild ☐ Cold BM Pressure: _____

☐ Dry ☐ Humid ☐ Wet Allergen Levels: _____

STRESS LEVELS

None	Low	Medium	High	Max	@$#%!

FOOD / MEDICATIONS

FOOD / DRINKS	MEDS / SUPPLEMENTS	TIME	DOSE

☐ usual daily medication

EXERCISE / DAILY ACTIVITY

☐ Heck yes, I worked out.

☐ I managed to exercise a bit.

☐ No, I haven't exercised at all.

☐ I did some stuff, and that counts.

DETAILS

NOTES / TRIGGERS / IMPROVEMENTS

_____

_____

_____

WRITE ONE THING YOU'RE GRATEFUL FOR

_____

*Date:*_____

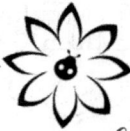

How are you feeling today?

| Like death | Terrible | Not good | Meh | Good | Great! | Amazing! |

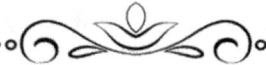

RATE YOUR PAIN LEVEL

① ② ③ ④ ⑤ ⑥ ⑦ ⑧ ⑨ ⑩

Describe your pain / symptoms

	am	pm
	☐	☐
	☐	☐
	☐	☐
	☐	☐
	☐	☐
	☐	☐
	☐	☐
	☐	☐

Where do you feel it?

Front   *Back*

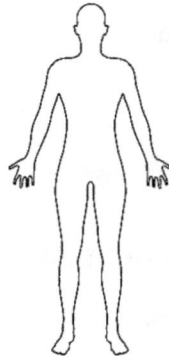
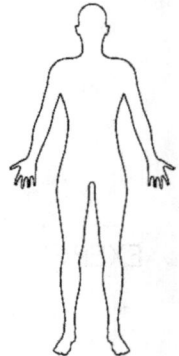

What about your...?

Mood	① ② ③ ④ ⑤ ⑥ ⑦ ⑧ ⑨ ⑩
Energy levels	① ② ③ ④ ⑤ ⑥ ⑦ ⑧ ⑨ ⑩
Mental clarity	① ② ③ ④ ⑤ ⑥ ⑦ ⑧ ⑨ ⑩

Feeling sick?

☐ Nope!

☐ Yes...

☐ Nausea   ☐ Diarrhea   ☐ Vomiting   ☐ Sore throat

☐ Congestion   ☐ Coughing   ☐ Chills   ☐ Fever

Other symptoms: _____

LET'S EXPLORE SOME MORE #45

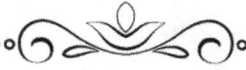

Hours of Sleep	① ② ③ ④ ⑤ ⑥ ⑦ ⑧ ⑨ ⑩ ⊕
Sleep Quality	① ② ③ ④ ⑤ ⑥ ⑦ ⑧ ⑨ ⑩

WEATHER

☐ Hot   ☐ Mild   ☐ Cold   BM Pressure: _____

☐ Dry   ☐ Humid   ☐ Wet   Allergen Levels: _____

STRESS LEVELS

None	Low	Medium	High	Max	@$#%!

FOOD / MEDICATIONS

FOOD / DRINKS	MEDS / SUPPLEMENTS	TIME	DOSE
	☐ usual daily medication		

EXERCISE / DAILY ACTIVITY

☐ Heck yes, I worked out.

☐ I managed to exercise a bit.

☐ No, I haven't exercised at all.

☐ I did some stuff, and that counts.

DETAILS

NOTES / TRIGGERS / IMPROVEMENTS

_____

_____

_____

WRITE ONE THING YOU'RE GRATEFUL FOR

_____

Date: _____

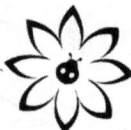

How are you feeling today?

Like death	Terrible	Not good	Meh	Good	Great!	Amazing!

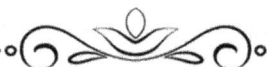

RATE YOUR PAIN LEVEL

(1) (2) (3) (4) (5) (6) (7) (8) (9) (10)

Describe your pain / symptoms

	am	pm
	☐	☐
	☐	☐
	☐	☐
	☐	☐
	☐	☐
	☐	☐
	☐	☐
	☐	☐

Where do you feel it?

Front   *Back*

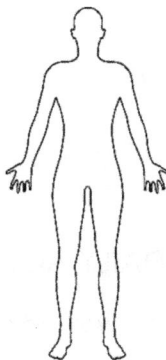

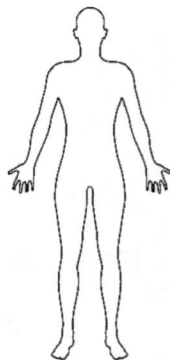

What about your...?

Mood	① ② ③ ④ ⑤ ⑥ ⑦ ⑧ ⑨ ⑩
Energy levels	① ② ③ ④ ⑤ ⑥ ⑦ ⑧ ⑨ ⑩
Mental clarity	① ② ③ ④ ⑤ ⑥ ⑦ ⑧ ⑨ ⑩

Feeling sick?

☐ Nope!

☐ Yes...

☐ Nausea ☐ Diarrhea ☐ Vomiting ☐ Sore throat

☐ Congestion ☐ Coughing ☐ Chills ☐ Fever

Other symptoms: _____

LET'S EXPLORE SOME MORE #46

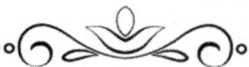

Hours of Sleep ① ② ③ ④ ⑤ ⑥ ⑦ ⑧ ⑨ ⑩ ⊕

Sleep Quality ① ② ③ ④ ⑤ ⑥ ⑦ ⑧ ⑨ ⑩

WEATHER

☐ Hot ☐ Mild ☐ Cold BM Pressure: _____

☐ Dry ☐ Humid ☐ Wet Allergen Levels: _____

STRESS LEVELS

| None | Low | Medium | High | Max | @$#%! |

FOOD / MEDICATIONS

FOOD / DRINKS	MEDS / SUPPLEMENTS	TIME	DOSE

☐ usual daily medication

EXERCISE / DAILY ACTIVITY

☐ Heck yes, I worked out.

☐ I managed to exercise a bit.

☐ No, I haven't exercised at all.

☐ I did some stuff, and that counts.

DETAILS

NOTES / TRIGGERS / IMPROVEMENTS

WRITE ONE THING YOU'RE GRATEFUL FOR

Date: _____

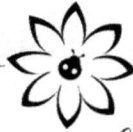

How are you feeling today?

Like death	Terrible	Not good	Meh	Good	Great!	Amazing!

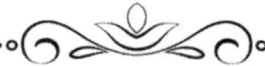

RATE YOUR PAIN LEVEL

① ② ③ ④ ⑤ ⑥ ⑦ ⑧ ⑨ ⑩

Describe your pain / symptoms

	am	pm
	☐	☐
	☐	☐
	☐	☐
	☐	☐
	☐	☐
	☐	☐
	☐	☐
	☐	☐

Where do you feel it?

Front   *Back*

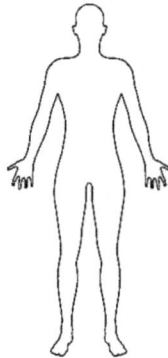

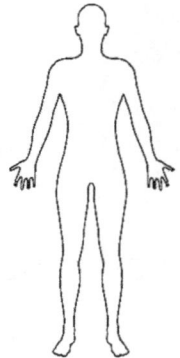

What about your...?

Mood	① ② ③ ④ ⑤ ⑥ ⑦ ⑧ ⑨ ⑩
Energy levels	① ② ③ ④ ⑤ ⑥ ⑦ ⑧ ⑨ ⑩
Mental clarity	① ② ③ ④ ⑤ ⑥ ⑦ ⑧ ⑨ ⑩

Feeling sick?

☐ Nope!
☐ Yes...

☐ Nausea ☐ Diarrhea ☐ Vomiting ☐ Sore throat

☐ Congestion ☐ Coughing ☐ Chills ☐ Fever

Other symptoms: _____

LET'S EXPLORE SOME MORE #47

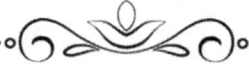

| Hours of Sleep | ① ② ③ ④ ⑤ ⑥ ⑦ ⑧ ⑨ ⑩ ⊕ |
| Sleep Quality | ① ② ③ ④ ⑤ ⑥ ⑦ ⑧ ⑨ ⑩ |

WEATHER

☐ Hot   ☐ Mild   ☐ Cold   BM Pressure: _____

☐ Dry   ☐ Humid   ☐ Wet   Allergen Levels: _____

STRESS LEVELS

| None | Low | Medium | High | Max | @$#%! |

FOOD / MEDICATIONS

FOOD / DRINKS	MEDS / SUPPLEMENTS	TIME	DOSE

☐ usual daily medication

EXERCISE / DAILY ACTIVITY

☐ Heck yes, I worked out.

☐ I managed to exercise a bit.

☐ No, I haven't exercised at all.

☐ I did some stuff, and that counts.

DETAILS

NOTES / TRIGGERS / IMPROVEMENTS

_____

_____

_____

WRITE ONE THING YOU'RE GRATEFUL FOR

_____

Date:_____

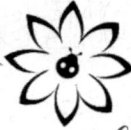

How are you feeling today?

😖	😣	😠	🙂	😊	😁	😍
Like death	Terrible	Not good	Meh	Good	Great!	Amazing!

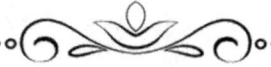

RATE YOUR PAIN LEVEL

① ② ③ ④ ⑤ ⑥ ⑦ ⑧ ⑨ ⑩

Describe your pain / symptoms

	am	pm
	☐	☐
	☐	☐
	☐	☐
	☐	☐
	☐	☐
	☐	☐
	☐	☐
	☐	☐

Where do you feel it?

Front   *Back*

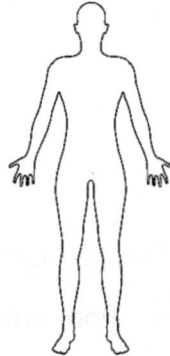

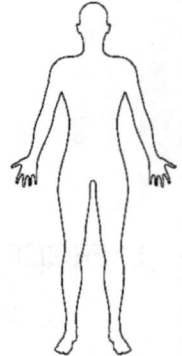

What about your...?

Mood	① ② ③ ④ ⑤ ⑥ ⑦ ⑧ ⑨ ⑩
Energy levels	① ② ③ ④ ⑤ ⑥ ⑦ ⑧ ⑨ ⑩
Mental clarity	① ② ③ ④ ⑤ ⑥ ⑦ ⑧ ⑨ ⑩

Feeling sick?

☐ Nope!
☐ Yes...

☐ Nausea   ☐ Diarrhea   ☐ Vomiting   ☐ Sore throat
☐ Congestion   ☐ Coughing   ☐ Chills   ☐ Fever

Other symptoms: _____

LET'S EXPLORE SOME MORE #48

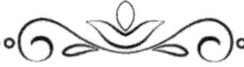

Hours of Sleep ① ② ③ ④ ⑤ ⑥ ⑦ ⑧ ⑨ ⑩ ⊕

Sleep Quality ① ② ③ ④ ⑤ ⑥ ⑦ ⑧ ⑨ ⑩

WEATHER

☐ Hot   ☐ Mild   ☐ Cold   BM Pressure: _____

☐ Dry   ☐ Humid   ☐ Wet   Allergen Levels: _____

STRESS LEVELS

None	Low	Medium	High	Max	@$#%!

FOOD / MEDICATIONS

FOOD / DRINKS	MEDS / SUPPLEMENTS	TIME	DOSE
	☐ usual daily medication		

EXERCISE / DAILY ACTIVITY

☐ Heck yes, I worked out.

☐ I managed to exercise a bit.

☐ No, I haven't exercised at all.

☐ I did some stuff, and that counts.

DETAILS

NOTES / TRIGGERS / IMPROVEMENTS

_____

_____

_____

WRITE ONE THING YOU'RE GRATEFUL FOR

_____

Date: _____

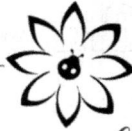

How are you feeling today?

Like death	Terrible	Not good	Meh	Good	Great!	Amazing!

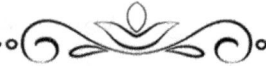

RATE YOUR PAIN LEVEL

① ② ③ ④ ⑤ ⑥ ⑦ ⑧ ⑨ ⑩

Describe your pain / symptoms

Where do you feel it?

am	pm
☐	☐
☐	☐
☐	☐
☐	☐
☐	☐
☐	☐
☐	☐
☐	☐

Front   *Back*

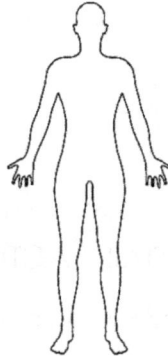

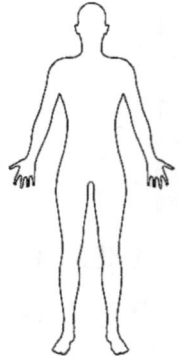

What about your...?

Feeling sick?

Mood ① ② ③ ④ ⑤ ⑥ ⑦ ⑧ ⑨ ⑩   ☐ Nope!

Energy levels ① ② ③ ④ ⑤ ⑥ ⑦ ⑧ ⑨ ⑩   ☐ Yes...

Mental clarity ① ② ③ ④ ⑤ ⑥ ⑦ ⑧ ⑨ ⑩

☐ Nausea   ☐ Diarrhea   ☐ Vomiting   ☐ Sore throat

☐ Congestion   ☐ Coughing   ☐ Chills   ☐ Fever

Other symptoms: _____

LET'S EXPLORE SOME MORE #49

Hours of Sleep ① ② ③ ④ ⑤ ⑥ ⑦ ⑧ ⑨ ⑩ ⊕

Sleep Quality ① ② ③ ④ ⑤ ⑥ ⑦ ⑧ ⑨ ⑩

WEATHER

☐ Hot ☐ Mild ☐ Cold BM Pressure: _____

☐ Dry ☐ Humid ☐ Wet Allergen Levels: _____

STRESS LEVELS

None	Low	Medium	High	Max	@$#%!

FOOD / MEDICATIONS

FOOD / DRINKS	MEDS / SUPPLEMENTS	TIME	DOSE

☐ usual daily medication

EXERCISE / DAILY ACTIVITY

☐ Heck yes, I worked out.

☐ I managed to exercise a bit.

☐ No, I haven't exercised at all.

☐ I did some stuff, and that counts.

DETAILS

NOTES / TRIGGERS / IMPROVEMENTS

_____

_____

_____

WRITE ONE THING YOU'RE GRATEFUL FOR

_____

Date:_____

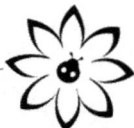

How are you feeling today?

Like death	Terrible	Not good	Meh	Good	Great!	Amazing!

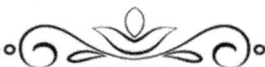

RATE YOUR PAIN LEVEL

① ② ③ ④ ⑤ ⑥ ⑦ ⑧ ⑨ ⑩

Describe your pain / symptoms

	am	pm
_____	☐	☐
_____	☐	☐
_____	☐	☐
_____	☐	☐
_____	☐	☐
_____	☐	☐
_____	☐	☐
_____	☐	☐

Where do you feel it?

Front   *Back*

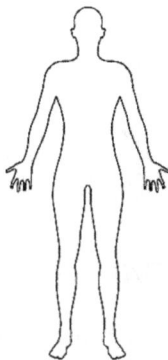

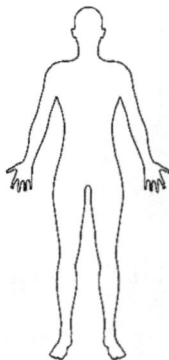

What about your...?

Mood	① ② ③ ④ ⑤ ⑥ ⑦ ⑧ ⑨ ⑩
Energy levels	① ② ③ ④ ⑤ ⑥ ⑦ ⑧ ⑨ ⑩
Mental clarity	① ② ③ ④ ⑤ ⑥ ⑦ ⑧ ⑨ ⑩

Feeling sick?

☐ Nope!
☐ Yes...

☐ Nausea   ☐ Diarrhea   ☐ Vomiting   ☐ Sore throat
☐ Congestion ☐ Coughing   ☐ Chills   ☐ Fever

Other symptoms: _____

LET'S EXPLORE SOME MORE #50

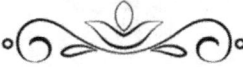

Hours of Sleep ① ② ③ ④ ⑤ ⑥ ⑦ ⑧ ⑨ ⑩ ⊕

Sleep Quality ① ② ③ ④ ⑤ ⑥ ⑦ ⑧ ⑨ ⑩

WEATHER

☐ Hot　☐ Mild　☐ Cold　BM Pressure: _____

☐ Dry　☐ Humid　☐ Wet　Allergen Levels: _____

STRESS LEVELS

None	Low	Medium	High	Max	@$#%!

FOOD / MEDICATIONS

FOOD / DRINKS	MEDS / SUPPLEMENTS	TIME	DOSE

☐ usual daily medication

EXERCISE / DAILY ACTIVITY

☐ Heck yes, I worked out.

☐ I managed to exercise a bit.

☐ No, I haven't exercised at all.

☐ I did some stuff, and that counts.

DETAILS

NOTES / TRIGGERS / IMPROVEMENTS

WRITE ONE THING YOU'RE GRATEFUL FOR

Date: _____

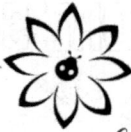

How are you feeling today?

| Like death | Terrible | Not good | Meh | Good | Great! | Amazing! |

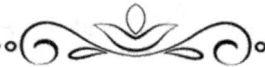

RATE YOUR PAIN LEVEL

(1) (2) (3) (4) (5) (6) (7) (8) (9) (10)

Describe your pain / symptoms

Where do you feel it?

	am	pm
_____	☐	☐
_____	☐	☐
_____	☐	☐
_____	☐	☐
_____	☐	☐
_____	☐	☐
_____	☐	☐
_____	☐	☐

Front   *Back*

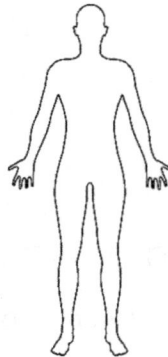 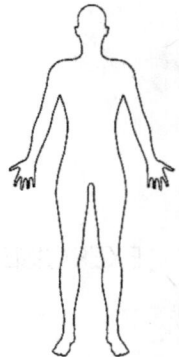

What about your...?

Feeling sick?

Mood   (1) (2) (3) (4) (5) (6) (7) (8) (9) (10)   ☐ Nope!

Energy levels   (1) (2) (3) (4) (5) (6) (7) (8) (9) (10)   ☐ Yes...

Mental clarity   (1) (2) (3) (4) (5) (6) (7) (8) (9) (10)

| ☐ Nausea | ☐ Diarrhea | ☐ Vomiting | ☐ Sore throat |
| ☐ Congestion | ☐ Coughing | ☐ Chills | ☐ Fever |

Other symptoms: _____

LET'S EXPLORE SOME MORE   #51

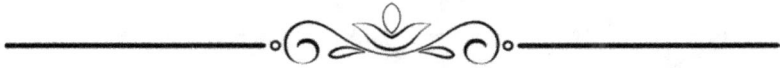

Hours of Sleep ① ② ③ ④ ⑤ ⑥ ⑦ ⑧ ⑨ ⑩ ⊕

Sleep Quality ① ② ③ ④ ⑤ ⑥ ⑦ ⑧ ⑨ ⑩

WEATHER

☐ Hot   ☐ Mild   ☐ Cold   BM Pressure: _____

☐ Dry   ☐ Humid   ☐ Wet   Allergen Levels: _____

STRESS LEVELS

None	Low	Medium	High	Max	@$#%!

FOOD / MEDICATIONS

FOOD / DRINKS	MEDS / SUPPLEMENTS	TIME	DOSE

☐ usual daily medication

EXERCISE / DAILY ACTIVITY

☐ Heck yes, I worked out.

☐ I managed to exercise a bit.

☐ No, I haven't exercised at all.

☐ I did some stuff, and that counts.

DETAILS

NOTES / TRIGGERS / IMPROVEMENTS

WRITE ONE THING YOU'RE GRATEFUL FOR

Date: _____

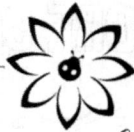

How are you feeling today?

| Like death | Terrible | Not good | Meh | Good | Great! | Amazing! |

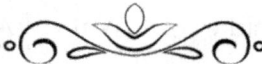

RATE YOUR PAIN LEVEL

(1) (2) (3) (4) (5) (6) (7) (8) (9) (10)

Describe your pain / symptoms

	am	pm
_____	☐	☐
_____	☐	☐
_____	☐	☐
_____	☐	☐
_____	☐	☐
_____	☐	☐
_____	☐	☐
_____	☐	☐

Where do you feel it?

Front   *Back*

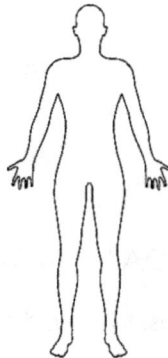

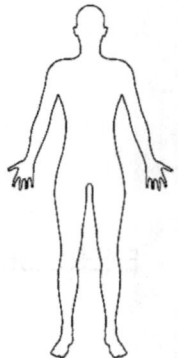

What about your...?

Mood	(1)	(2)	(3)	(4)	(5)	(6)	(7)	(8)	(9)	(10)
Energy levels	(1)	(2)	(3)	(4)	(5)	(6)	(7)	(8)	(9)	(10)
Mental clarity	(1)	(2)	(3)	(4)	(5)	(6)	(7)	(8)	(9)	(10)

Feeling sick?

☐ Nope!

☐ Yes...

☐ Nausea   ☐ Diarrhea   ☐ Vomiting   ☐ Sore throat

☐ Congestion   ☐ Coughing   ☐ Chills   ☐ Fever

Other symptoms: _____

LET'S EXPLORE SOME MORE #52

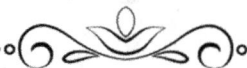

Hours of Sleep ① ② ③ ④ ⑤ ⑥ ⑦ ⑧ ⑨ ⑩ ⊕
Sleep Quality ① ② ③ ④ ⑤ ⑥ ⑦ ⑧ ⑨ ⑩

WEATHER

☐ Hot ☐ Mild ☐ Cold BM Pressure: _____

☐ Dry ☐ Humid ☐ Wet Allergen Levels: _____

STRESS LEVELS

None	Low	Medium	High	Max	@$#%!

FOOD / MEDICATIONS

FOOD / DRINKS	MEDS / SUPPLEMENTS	TIME	DOSE

☐ usual daily medication

EXERCISE / DAILY ACTIVITY

☐ Heck yes, I worked out.

☐ I managed to exercise a bit.

☐ No, I haven't exercised at all.

☐ I did some stuff, and that counts.

DETAILS

NOTES / TRIGGERS / IMPROVEMENTS

WRITE ONE THING YOU'RE GRATEFUL FOR

Date:_____

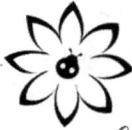

How are you feeling today?

Like death	Terrible	Not good	Meh	Good	Great!	Amazing!

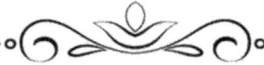

RATE YOUR PAIN LEVEL

① ② ③ ④ ⑤ ⑥ ⑦ ⑧ ⑨ ⑩

Describe your pain / symptoms

	am	pm
	☐	☐
	☐	☐
	☐	☐
	☐	☐
	☐	☐
	☐	☐
	☐	☐
	☐	☐

Where do you feel it?

Front   *Back*

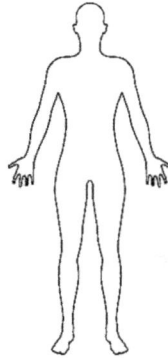

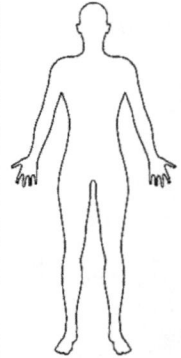

What about your...?

Mood	① ② ③ ④ ⑤ ⑥ ⑦ ⑧ ⑨ ⑩
Energy levels	① ② ③ ④ ⑤ ⑥ ⑦ ⑧ ⑨ ⑩
Mental clarity	① ② ③ ④ ⑤ ⑥ ⑦ ⑧ ⑨ ⑩

Feeling sick?

☐ Nope!
☐ Yes...

☐ Nausea   ☐ Diarrhea   ☐ Vomiting   ☐ Sore throat
☐ Congestion   ☐ Coughing   ☐ Chills   ☐ Fever

Other symptoms:_____

LET'S EXPLORE SOME MORE #53

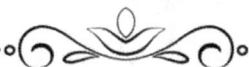

Hours of Sleep ① ② ③ ④ ⑤ ⑥ ⑦ ⑧ ⑨ ⑩ ⊕

Sleep Quality ① ② ③ ④ ⑤ ⑥ ⑦ ⑧ ⑨ ⑩

WEATHER

☐ Hot ☐ Mild ☐ Cold BM Pressure: _____

☐ Dry ☐ Humid ☐ Wet Allergen Levels: _____

STRESS LEVELS

None	Low	Medium	High	Max	@$#%!

FOOD / MEDICATIONS

FOOD / DRINKS	MEDS / SUPPLEMENTS	TIME	DOSE

☐ usual daily medication

EXERCISE / DAILY ACTIVITY

☐ Heck yes, I worked out.

☐ I managed to exercise a bit.

☐ No, I haven't exercised at all.

☐ I did some stuff, and that counts.

DETAILS

NOTES / TRIGGERS / IMPROVEMENTS

WRITE ONE THING YOU'RE GRATEFUL FOR

Date:_____

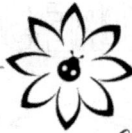

How are you feeling today?

Like death	Terrible	Not good	Meh	Good	Great!	Amazing!

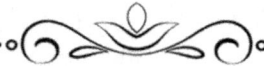

RATE YOUR PAIN LEVEL

(1) (2) (3) (4) (5) (6) (7) (8) (9) (10)

Describe your pain / symptoms   Where do you feel it?

	am	pm		Front	Back
	☐	☐			
	☐	☐			
	☐	☐			
	☐	☐			
	☐	☐			
	☐	☐			
	☐	☐			
	☐	☐			

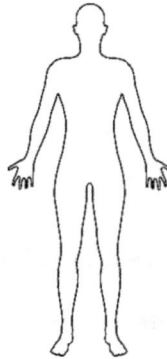

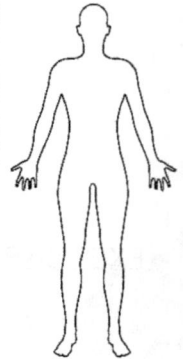

What about your...?   Feeling sick?

Mood   (1) (2) (3) (4) (5) (6) (7) (8) (9) (10)   ☐ Nope!

Energy levels   (1) (2) (3) (4) (5) (6) (7) (8) (9) (10)   ☐ Yes...

Mental clarity (1) (2) (3) (4) (5) (6) (7) (8) (9) (10)

☐ Nausea   ☐ Diarrhea   ☐ Vomiting   ☐ Sore throat

☐ Congestion ☐ Coughing   ☐ Chills   ☐ Fever

Other symptoms: _____

LET'S EXPLORE SOME MORE #54

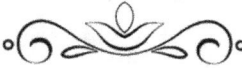

| Hours of Sleep | ① ② ③ ④ ⑤ ⑥ ⑦ ⑧ ⑨ ⑩ ⊕ |
| Sleep Quality | ① ② ③ ④ ⑤ ⑥ ⑦ ⑧ ⑨ ⑩ |

WEATHER

☐ Hot ☐ Mild ☐ Cold BM Pressure: _____

☐ Dry ☐ Humid ☐ Wet Allergen Levels: _____

STRESS LEVELS

| None | Low | Medium | High | Max | @$#%! |

FOOD / MEDICATIONS

FOOD / DRINKS	MEDS / SUPPLEMENTS	TIME	DOSE
	☐ usual daily medication		

EXERCISE / DAILY ACTIVITY

☐ Heck yes, I worked out.

☐ I managed to exercise a bit.

☐ No, I haven't exercised at all.

☐ I did some stuff, and that counts.

DETAILS

NOTES / TRIGGERS / IMPROVEMENTS

_____

_____

_____

WRITE ONE THING YOU'RE GRATEFUL FOR

_____

Date: _____

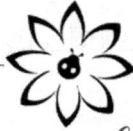

How are you feeling today?

| Like death | Terrible | Not good | Meh | Good | Great! | Amazing! |

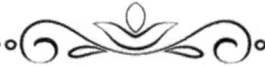

RATE YOUR PAIN LEVEL

① ② ③ ④ ⑤ ⑥ ⑦ ⑧ ⑨ ⑩

Describe your pain / symptoms

Where do you feel it?

	am	pm
_____	☐	☐
_____	☐	☐
_____	☐	☐
_____	☐	☐
_____	☐	☐
_____	☐	☐
_____	☐	☐
_____	☐	☐

Front   *Back*

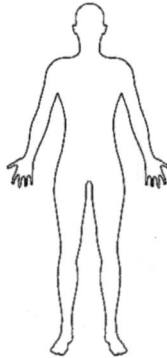

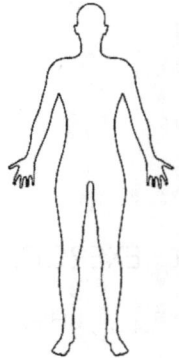

What about your...?

Feeling sick?

Mood	① ② ③ ④ ⑤ ⑥ ⑦ ⑧ ⑨ ⑩	☐ Nope!
Energy levels	① ② ③ ④ ⑤ ⑥ ⑦ ⑧ ⑨ ⑩	☐ Yes...
Mental clarity	① ② ③ ④ ⑤ ⑥ ⑦ ⑧ ⑨ ⑩	

☐ Nausea   ☐ Diarrhea   ☐ Vomiting   ☐ Sore throat

☐ Congestion   ☐ Coughing   ☐ Chills   ☐ Fever

Other symptoms: _____

LET'S EXPLORE SOME MORE #55

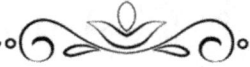

Hours of Sleep (1) (2) (3) (4) (5) (6) (7) (8) (9) (10) (+)

Sleep Quality (1) (2) (3) (4) (5) (6) (7) (8) (9) (10)

WEATHER

☐ Hot ☐ Mild ☐ Cold BM Pressure: _____

☐ Dry ☐ Humid ☐ Wet Allergen Levels: _____

STRESS LEVELS

None	Low	Medium	High	Max	@$#%!

FOOD / MEDICATIONS

FOOD / DRINKS	MEDS / SUPPLEMENTS	TIME	DOSE

☐ usual daily medication

EXERCISE / DAILY ACTIVITY

☐ Heck yes, I worked out.

☐ I managed to exercise a bit.

☐ No, I haven't exercised at all.

☐ I did some stuff, and that counts.

DETAILS

NOTES / TRIGGERS / IMPROVEMENTS

_____

_____

_____

WRITE ONE THING YOU'RE GRATEFUL FOR

_____

Date: _____

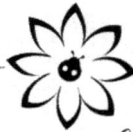

How are you feeling today?

Like death	Terrible	Not good	Meh	Good	Great!	Amazing!

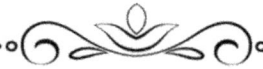

RATE YOUR PAIN LEVEL

(1) (2) (3) (4) (5) (6) (7) (8) (9) (10)

Describe your pain / symptoms   Where do you feel it?

	am	pm
	☐	☐
	☐	☐
	☐	☐
	☐	☐
	☐	☐
	☐	☐
	☐	☐
	☐	☐

Front   Back

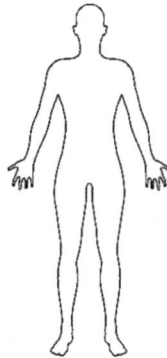

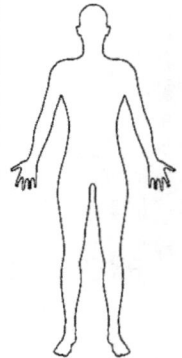

What about your...?   Feeling sick?

Mood   ① ② ③ ④ ⑤ ⑥ ⑦ ⑧ ⑨ ⑩   ☐ Nope!

Energy levels   ① ② ③ ④ ⑤ ⑥ ⑦ ⑧ ⑨ ⑩   ☐ Yes...

Mental clarity ① ② ③ ④ ⑤ ⑥ ⑦ ⑧ ⑨ ⑩

☐ Nausea   ☐ Diarrhea   ☐ Vomiting   ☐ Sore throat

☐ Congestion   ☐ Coughing   ☐ Chills   ☐ Fever

Other symptoms: _____

LET'S EXPLORE SOME MORE #56

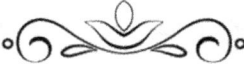

Hours of Sleep ① ② ③ ④ ⑤ ⑥ ⑦ ⑧ ⑨ ⑩ ⊕

Sleep Quality ① ② ③ ④ ⑤ ⑥ ⑦ ⑧ ⑨ ⑩

WEATHER

☐ Hot ☐ Mild ☐ Cold BM Pressure: _____

☐ Dry ☐ Humid ☐ Wet Allergen Levels: _____

STRESS LEVELS

| None | Low | Medium | High | Max | @$#%! |

FOOD / MEDICATIONS

FOOD / DRINKS	MEDS / SUPPLEMENTS	TIME	DOSE

☐ usual daily medication

EXERCISE / DAILY ACTIVITY

☐ Heck yes, I worked out.

☐ I managed to exercise a bit.

☐ No, I haven't exercised at all.

☐ I did some stuff, and that counts.

DETAILS

NOTES / TRIGGERS / IMPROVEMENTS

_____

_____

_____

WRITE ONE THING YOU'RE GRATEFUL FOR

_____

Date:_____

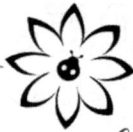

How are you feeling today?

😵 Like death   😣 Terrible   ☹️ Not good   🙂 Meh   😃 Good   😁 Great!   🥰 Amazing!

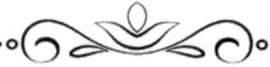

RATE YOUR PAIN LEVEL

① ② ③ ④ ⑤ ⑥ ⑦ ⑧ ⑨ ⑩

Describe your pain / symptoms

	am	pm
	☐	☐
	☐	☐
	☐	☐
	☐	☐
	☐	☐
	☐	☐
	☐	☐
	☐	☐

Where do you feel it?

Front   *Back*

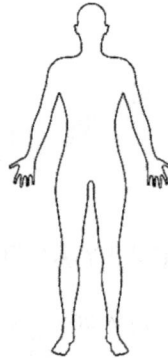 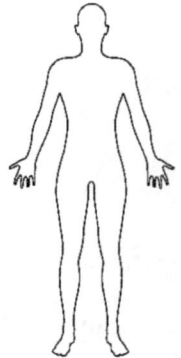

What about your...?

Mood   ① ② ③ ④ ⑤ ⑥ ⑦ ⑧ ⑨ ⑩
Energy levels ① ② ③ ④ ⑤ ⑥ ⑦ ⑧ ⑨ ⑩
Mental clarity ① ② ③ ④ ⑤ ⑥ ⑦ ⑧ ⑨ ⑩

Feeling sick?

☐ Nope!
☐ Yes...

☐ Nausea   ☐ Diarrhea   ☐ Vomiting   ☐ Sore throat
☐ Congestion ☐ Coughing   ☐ Chills   ☐ Fever

Other symptoms:

LET'S EXPLORE SOME MORE #57

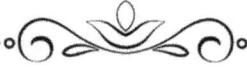

Hours of Sleep ① ② ③ ④ ⑤ ⑥ ⑦ ⑧ ⑨ ⑩ ⊕

Sleep Quality ① ② ③ ④ ⑤ ⑥ ⑦ ⑧ ⑨ ⑩

WEATHER

☐ Hot ☐ Mild ☐ Cold   BM Pressure: _____

☐ Dry ☐ Humid ☐ Wet   Allergen Levels: _____

STRESS LEVELS

| None | Low | Medium | High | Max | @$#%! |

FOOD / MEDICATIONS

FOOD / DRINKS	MEDS / SUPPLEMENTS	TIME	DOSE

☐ usual daily medication

EXERCISE / DAILY ACTIVITY

☐ Heck yes, I worked out.

☐ I managed to exercise a bit.

☐ No, I haven't exercised at all.

☐ I did some stuff, and that counts.

DETAILS

NOTES / TRIGGERS / IMPROVEMENTS

_____

_____

_____

WRITE ONE THING YOU'RE GRATEFUL FOR

_____

Date:_____

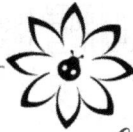

How are you feeling today?

Like death	Terrible	Not good	Meh	Good	Great!	Amazing!

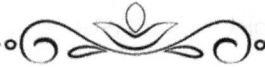

RATE YOUR PAIN LEVEL

① ② ③ ④ ⑤ ⑥ ⑦ ⑧ ⑨ ⑩

Describe your pain / symptoms   Where do you feel it?

	am	pm
	☐	☐
	☐	☐
	☐	☐
	☐	☐
	☐	☐
	☐	☐
	☐	☐
	☐	☐

Front   *Back*

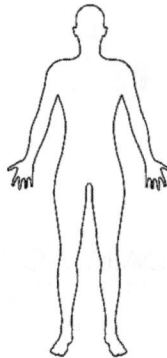

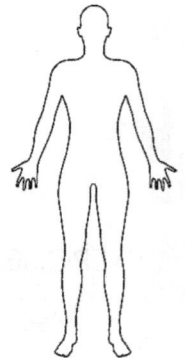

What about your...?   Feeling sick?

Mood	① ② ③ ④ ⑤ ⑥ ⑦ ⑧ ⑨ ⑩	☐ Nope!
Energy levels	① ② ③ ④ ⑤ ⑥ ⑦ ⑧ ⑨ ⑩	☐ Yes...
Mental clarity	① ② ③ ④ ⑤ ⑥ ⑦ ⑧ ⑨ ⑩	

☐ Nausea   ☐ Diarrhea   ☐ Vomiting   ☐ Sore throat

☐ Congestion   ☐ Coughing   ☐ Chills   ☐ Fever

Other symptoms: _____

LET'S EXPLORE SOME MORE #58

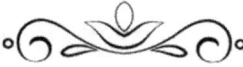

Hours of Sleep ① ② ③ ④ ⑤ ⑥ ⑦ ⑧ ⑨ ⑩ ⊕
Sleep Quality ① ② ③ ④ ⑤ ⑥ ⑦ ⑧ ⑨ ⑩

WEATHER

☐ Hot   ☐ Mild   ☐ Cold   BM Pressure: _____
☐ Dry   ☐ Humid   ☐ Wet   Allergen Levels: _____

STRESS LEVELS

| None | Low | Medium | High | Max | @$#%! |

FOOD / MEDICATIONS

FOOD / DRINKS	MEDS / SUPPLEMENTS	TIME	DOSE

☐ usual daily medication

EXERCISE / DAILY ACTIVITY

☐ Heck yes, I worked out.
☐ I managed to exercise a bit.
☐ No, I haven't exercised at all.
☐ I did some stuff, and that counts.

DETAILS

NOTES / TRIGGERS / IMPROVEMENTS

WRITE ONE THING YOU'RE GRATEFUL FOR

Date:_____

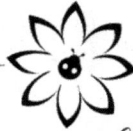

How are you feeling today?

Like death	Terrible	Not good	Meh	Good	Great!	Amazing!

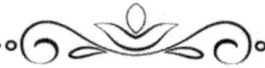

RATE YOUR PAIN LEVEL

① ② ③ ④ ⑤ ⑥ ⑦ ⑧ ⑨ ⑩

Describe your pain / symptoms

Where do you feel it?

am	pm
☐	☐
☐	☐
☐	☐
☐	☐
☐	☐
☐	☐
☐	☐
☐	☐

Front   *Back*

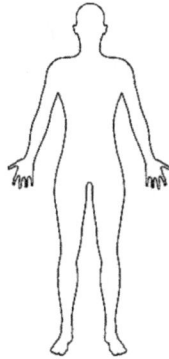

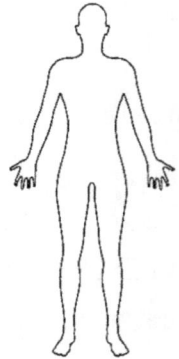

What about your...?

Feeling sick?

Mood ① ② ③ ④ ⑤ ⑥ ⑦ ⑧ ⑨ ⑩   ☐ Nope!

Energy levels ① ② ③ ④ ⑤ ⑥ ⑦ ⑧ ⑨ ⑩   ☐ Yes...

Mental clarity ① ② ③ ④ ⑤ ⑥ ⑦ ⑧ ⑨ ⑩

☐ Nausea   ☐ Diarrhea   ☐ Vomiting   ☐ Sore throat

☐ Congestion   ☐ Coughing   ☐ Chills   ☐ Fever

Other symptoms:_____

LET'S EXPLORE SOME MORE #59

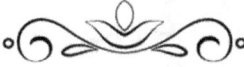

Hours of Sleep (1) (2) (3) (4) (5) (6) (7) (8) (9) (10) (+)

Sleep Quality (1) (2) (3) (4) (5) (6) (7) (8) (9) (10)

WEATHER

☐ Hot   ☐ Mild   ☐ Cold   BM Pressure: _____

☐ Dry   ☐ Humid   ☐ Wet   Allergen Levels: _____

STRESS LEVELS

None	Low	Medium	High	Max	@$#%!

FOOD / MEDICATIONS

FOOD / DRINKS	MEDS / SUPPLEMENTS	TIME	DOSE
	☐ usual daily medication		

EXERCISE / DAILY ACTIVITY

☐ Heck yes, I worked out.

☐ I managed to exercise a bit.

☐ No, I haven't exercised at all.

☐ I did some stuff, and that counts.

DETAILS

NOTES / TRIGGERS / IMPROVEMENTS

_____

_____

_____

WRITE ONE THING YOU'RE GRATEFUL FOR

_____

Date: _____

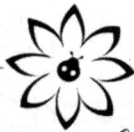

How are you feeling today?

| Like death | Terrible | Not good | Meh | Good | Great! | Amazing! |

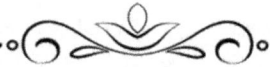

RATE YOUR PAIN LEVEL

(1) (2) (3) (4) (5) (6) (7) (8) (9) (10)

Describe your pain / symptoms   Where do you feel it?

	am	pm
	☐	☐
	☐	☐
	☐	☐
	☐	☐
	☐	☐
	☐	☐
	☐	☐
	☐	☐

Front   *Back*

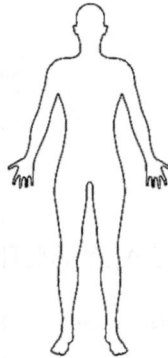 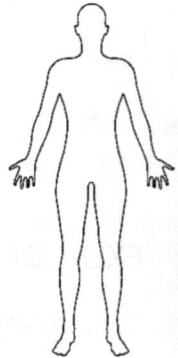

What about your...?   Feeling sick?

Mood   (1) (2) (3) (4) (5) (6) (7) (8) (9) (10)   ☐ Nope!

Energy levels (1) (2) (3) (4) (5) (6) (7) (8) (9) (10)   ☐ Yes...

Mental clarity (1) (2) (3) (4) (5) (6) (7) (8) (9) (10)

☐ Nausea   ☐ Diarrhea   ☐ Vomiting   ☐ Sore throat

☐ Congestion   ☐ Coughing   ☐ Chills   ☐ Fever

Other symptoms: _____

LET'S EXPLORE SOME MORE #60

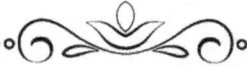

Hours of Sleep ① ② ③ ④ ⑤ ⑥ ⑦ ⑧ ⑨ ⑩ ⊕

Sleep Quality ① ② ③ ④ ⑤ ⑥ ⑦ ⑧ ⑨ ⑩

WEATHER

☐ Hot ☐ Mild ☐ Cold BM Pressure: _____

☐ Dry ☐ Humid ☐ Wet Allergen Levels: _____

STRESS LEVELS

None	Low	Medium	High	Max	@$#%!

FOOD / MEDICATIONS

FOOD / DRINKS	MEDS / SUPPLEMENTS	TIME	DOSE

☐ usual daily medication

EXERCISE / DAILY ACTIVITY

☐ Heck yes, I worked out.

☐ I managed to exercise a bit.

☐ No, I haven't exercised at all.

☐ I did some stuff, and that counts.

DETAILS

NOTES / TRIGGERS / IMPROVEMENTS

_____

_____

_____

WRITE ONE THING YOU'RE GRATEFUL FOR

_____

Notes

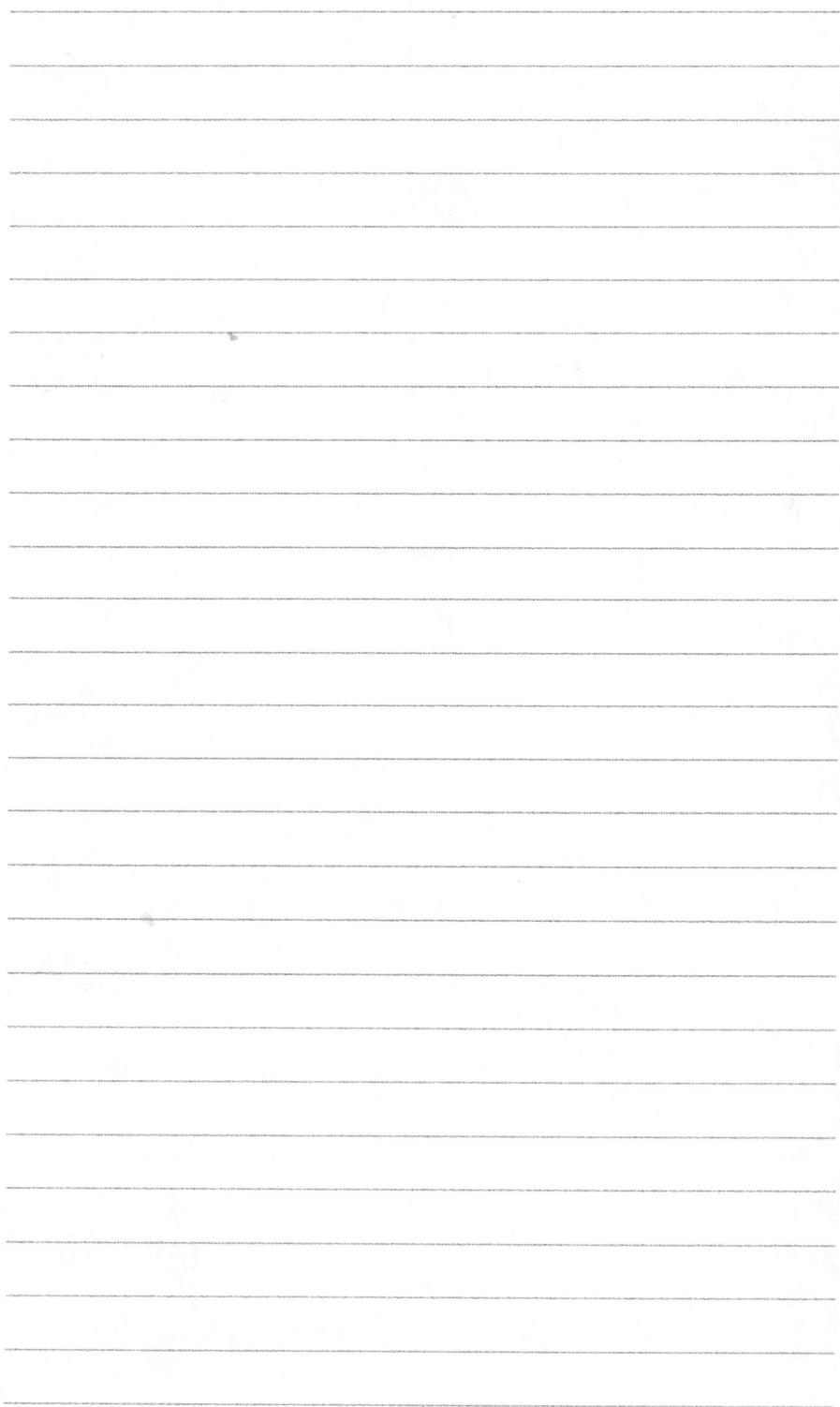

www.ingramcontent.com/pod-product-compliance
Lightning Source LLC
Chambersburg PA
CBHW051026030426
42336CB00015B/2741